Allergic Contact Dermatitis to Simple Chemicals

DERMATOLOGY

series editors

Charles D. Calnan

Consultant Dermatologist
University of London–British Postgraduate Medical Federation
St. John's Hospital for Diseases of the Skin
London, England

Howard I. Maibach

Department of Dermatology
University of California School of Medicine
Ambulatory Care Center 342
San Francisco, California

Additional Volumes in Preparation

Allergic Contact Dermatitis to Simple Chemicals

A MOLECULAR APPROACH

GILLES DUPUIS
Faculté de Médecine
Université de Sherbrooke
Sherbrooke, Canada

CLAUDE BENEZRA
Institut de Chimie
Université Louis Pasteur de Strasbourg
Strasbourg, France

MARCEL DEKKER, INC.   New York and Basel

Library of Congress Cataloging in Publication Data

Dupuis, Gilles, [date]
    Allergic contact dermatitis to simple chemicals.

    (Dermatology ; v. 2)
    Includes bibliographical references and indexes.
    1. Contact dermatitis. 2. Allergens.
I. Benezra, Claude. II. Title. III. Series:
Dermatology (Marcel Dekker, Inc.) ; v. 2. [DNLM:
1. Dermatitis, Contact. 2. Haptens—Classification.
W1 DE5084 v.2 / WR 175 D944a]
RC593.C6D86]982   616.97'307   82-10082
ISBN 0-8247-1468-7

MARCEL DEKKER, INC.
270 Madison Avenue, New York, New York 10016

Current printing (last digit):
10 9 8 7 6 5 4 3 2 1

PRINTED IN THE UNITED STATES OF AMERICA

This book is dedicated to

my parents, M. and Mme L. Dupuis, and to my wife, Patricia. −G.D.
my lovely daughters, Annouchka and Patricia. −C.B.

Introduction to the Series

Many dermatologists along with other doctors and scientists were surprised by the views of an eminent medical Nobel Prize winner who said that all the major discoveries in biology have been made and little can be expected from now on. The scientific achievements of the past 40 years, even in relation to medicine alone, have been so phenomenal that one may wonder if there is anything of importance left for future generations. The same attitude may be taken with regard to medical books, and especially in relation to dermatology. So much has been written over the past 30 years that one may question whether there are any books of value left to be written. Nothing could be further from the truth.

The functions of medical journals and medical books are different. As the number, diversity, and output of journals expands, so does the need for medical books; this is as true for dermatology as for any other branch of medicine. And it is equally true for the subdivisions of dermatology. Some doctors may regret increasing subspecialization within a single branch such as dermatology, but it is a reflection of the steady and inevitable increase in knowledge within the subject. Specialized clinics and departments are now the norm rather than the exception within many university dermatological centers. Their outward manifestation is the growth of subspecialty journals in relation to such subjects as dermatological surgery and oncology, contact dermatitis and occupational dermatoses, microbiology, and pediatric dermatology.

The subdivision of subjects such as dermatology today is a reflection of the subdivision of internal medicine 40 years ago, and it produces similar opposing groups of antagonists. The dearth of the general dermatologist may come to be mourned in the same way as has the dearth of the general physician. But the practical clinical dermatologist and the physician who has responsibility for the care of patients with skin disease will usually depend more on books than on journals when he/she needs help. This is particularly true of dermatologists who work away from university centers, especially outside Western Europe and North America, and who constitute a "silent majority." Although there is still a place for the comprehensive textbook, the growth of specialist books has shown the need for such condensation of recent specialist information.

The Medical Division of Marcel Dekker, Inc. has decided to meet this need with a selective series of books on particular branches of dermatology, especially in fields which have frontiers with more than one scientific discipline. The emphasis, however, will be on the information requirements of dermatologists whose responsibilities involve not only the clinical care of patients, but also extend to education and research.

Charles D. Calnan, M.D.
Howard Maibach, M.D.

Foreword

Some areas of science explode by the very nature of their pertinence and time-liness: genetic engineering and molecular biology are current examples. The basis of molecular approach to allergic contact dermatitis was laid down four decades ago by Landsteiner and his early followers; it has now come of age.

Drs. Dupuis and Benezra are the first to synthesize isolated advances over these decades and provide a working hypothesis for all interested in structure-function relationships in allergic contact dermatitis and related fields (the broader areas of cell-mediated or delayed hypersensitivity).

The first chapters offer entrance into the field for the novitiate, that is, a crisp summary of general knowledge of cell-mediated immunity. A brief review of toxicologic techniques utilized in animals and man provides insight into identifying potential contact allergies.

Chapter 5 offers a succinct and brilliantly clear explanation of the chemistry involved in bonding of simple chemical to the protein carrier. Chapter 6 details the chemically reactive functions in haptens and proteins. The authors also present an innovative—and certainly useful—classification of haptens according to "their medical reactivity in relationship to putative carrier protein." This lucid classification guarantees the wide quotation of this chapter for years to come.

Drs. Dupuis and Benezra next provide a theoretical basis for the concept of the prohapten: this explains how chemicals may be transformed into reactive moities, capable of acting as allergens.

The last chapter synthesizes our extensive, often fragmentary information on cross reactions into a comprehensible molecular overview.

What patient, physician, or dermatologist has not wondered why a chemical (poison ivy, neomycin, or an industrial agent) is an allergen? Now we have a theoretical framework—backed with extensive documentation—to begin to answer this question.

I predict that Drs. Dupuis and Benezra's book will provide the long overdue stimulus for much new work in this field which will be of great theoretical and practical benefit to human beings.

Howard Maibach
San Francisco

Preface

Allergic contact dermatitis (ACD) is a fairly common skin affliction. The
causative agents of this disease are of vastly different origins, ranging from
naturally occurring metabolites to synthetic dyes, drugs, and other chemicals.
Owing to the fact that a great many new chemicals appear every year on the
market, it may be expected that additional contact allergens will be added to
an already impressive list. We felt, therefore, that a classification of identified
allergens (haptens) was appropriate at this time. In this book we have attempted to give some general outlines that will serve to classify newly identified allergenic chemicals.

The book is organized into two major divisions. First, a brief review of
the cellular aspects of allergic contact dermatitis is presented (Chap. 1). A
description of the most common approaches used to study ACD in vitro
(Chap. 2) and in vivo (Chap. 3) follows. In Chapter 4, the concept of the
carrier in ACD is discussed. Chapter 5 introduces the second main theme of
the book—the chemical and structural aspects of ACD. In this chapter, the
basic chemical reactions in which allergens (haptens) and proteins (carriers)
can participate are reviewed briefly. This chapter is followed by a review
(Chapter 6) of the chemical properties of amino acid side chains and a classification of haptens based on the kinds of chemical reactions they can undergo. Chapter 7 examines the phenomenon of cross-sensitization, with an attempt to rationalize it from a structural standpoint, that is, by examination
of the structures of the chemicals implicated.

This book has been written with the purpose of attempting to understand

and rationalize ACD from a structural (chemical) point of view. For this reason, dermatologists, allergologists, biochemists, chemists, and any individual interested by the phenomenon of contact dermatitis may find this book a valuable tool.

The immunologic aspects of ACD are not dealt with in depth here. Readers can find a more complete description of this aspect in published books, review articles, and book series. In addition, primary irritations have not been considered because they do not appear to be the result of an immune reaction.

The authors do not pretend to offer a general explanation for the phenomeono of ACD; we simply propose an original classification of haptens involved in ACD. This classification may serve to predict the potential allergenicity of new chemicals.

We wish to thank the many persons and granting organizations that have made the work described in the authors' laboratories possible. In particular, our most sincere thanks are due to Drs. J. C. Mitchell and J. Foussereau for helpful and stimulating discussions. Financial support from the Conseil de Recherches Médicales du Canada, La Direction Générale de la Recherche Scientifique et Technologique, and Institut National de Santé et de Recherches Médicales is gratefully acknowledged. The patience of Ms. L. Bibeau made the typing of this work possible.

Finally, we take this opportunity to express our thanks to the many friends and collaborators which have contributed, by their support and advice, to this book.

G. Dupuis
C. Benezra

Contents

Allergic Contact Dermatitis to Simple Chemicals

1

Immunologic Aspects of Allergic Contact Dermatitis

Contact dermatitis caused by exposure to certain chemicals or plants has been known for many centuries. In 1840, the phenomenon was thought to be "selective": it was observed that some individuals developed reactions to certain external agents while others did not (Fuchs, 1840). Fuchs' observations were followed by intensive work using skin testing to most common chemicals (tincture of arnica, mercury salts, turpentine, soaps, etc.) (Hebra, 1869). Further progress in the study of allergic contact dermatitis (ACD) was accomplished by the technique of patch testing developed by Jadassohn (1895, 1896). Using this method, it became possible to investigate the nature of allergens responsible for ACD in sensitive subjects.

Chemical investigations of the nature of allergens along with clinical testing contributed to a gradual understanding of ACD. An important breakthrough occurred when it was shown that a concentrated ether extract of primrose leaves (*Primula*) could sensitize human subjects (Bloch and Steiner-Wourlisch 1926). Shortly thereafter it was observed that human volunteers could be sensitized to *p*-phenylenediamine (PPD) (Mayer, 1928). Other chemicals, such as 2,4-dinitrochlorobenzene (DNCB), which was used to induce contact dermatitis in man (Wedroff, 1927, 1932; Wedroff and Dolgoff, 1935), also proved to be valuable tools in the experimental study of ACD. An equally important step was the discovery that guinea pigs could serve as a model for the study of contact dermatitis (Bloch and Steiner-Wourlisch, 1930; Jadassohn, 1930).

Induction of ACD

The systematic work of Landsteiner and his group was the first direct approach
to study the mechanism of ACD. Chemicals possessing a very simple structure
such as benzene substituted with halogens, nitro groups, or both, were found
to possess sensitizing properties (in the guinea pig) only when the substituting
groups could be displaced by aniline (Landsteiner and Jacobs, 1936) (Table 1).
Landsteiner's results were further supported by findings from other groups.
For instance, it was shown that experimental results obtained with guinea pigs
sensitized with simple chemicals could be reproduced in man (Sulzberger and
Baer, 1938).

The initial concept that simple chemicals needed to possess one or more reactive group(s) was then put forward as a prerequisite for chemical induction
of sensitization. Hapten-protein conjugates were prepared by Landsteiner's
group, and it was shown that such adducts could induce sensitization in experimental animals and positive cutaneous reactions in animals sensitive to the
hapten. Landsteiner also obtained positive results using picryl chloride coupled
to red cell stromata (Landsteiner and Chase, 1941).

Other groups have further shown that haptens coupled to globulins or albumins (Benacerraf and Gell, 1959a, 1959b; Cohen, 1966; Gell and Benacerraf,
1961; Kruger et al., 1971; Ovary and Benacerraf, 1963), gelatin (Arnon and
Sela, 1960; Sela and Arnon, 1960), synthetic polymers of lysine (Schlossman
et al., 1965, 1966), serum proteins (Parker et al., 1970; Parker and turk, 1970),
or skin proteins (Dupuis, 1979; Dupuis et al., 1980; Milner, 1970, 1972; Nakagawa and Tanioku, 1972; Parker and Turk, 1970) can elicit sensitization or
positive reactions in experimental animals.

These results support Landsteiner's original concept that a simple chemical
molecule possessing a definite chemical reactivity forms, when coupled to a
carrier, a complete antigen capable of producing sensitization and ACD (Benacerraf and Levine, 1962; Borek and Stupp, 1965; Chase, 1966; Dupuis et al.,
1980; Eisen et al., 1952; Eisen and Belman, 1953; Eisen and Tabachnick, 1958;
Eisen et al., 1959; Eisen 1959; Gell and Benacerraf, 1961; Gell and Silverstein,
1962; Kantor et al., 1963; Medawar, 1965; Salvin and Smith, 1961; Silverstein
and Gell, 1962).

ACD and the Tuberculin Reaction

In the late nineteenth century, Koch showed that subcutaneous injection of
old tuberculin produces a severe general reaction associated with redness and
inflammation at the site of injection in tuberculous patients (Koch, 1890).

Table 1 Sensitizing Power of Some Substituted Benzene Derivatives

Substance	Reaction with aniline	Sensitization
1-Chloro-2,4-dinitrobenzene	+	positive
1-Bromo-2,4-dinitrobenzene	+	positive
1-Iodo-2,4-dinitrobenzene	+	positive
1-Fluoro-2,4-dinitrobenzene	+	positive
1,4-Dichloro-2,6-dinitrobenzene	+	positive
1,3-Dichloro-4,6-dinitrobenzene	+	positive
1-Chloro-2,4,6-trinitrobenzene	+	positive
1,3-Dichloro-5-nitrobenzene	–	negative
1,4-Dichloro-2-nitrobenzene	–	negative
1,2-Dichloro-4-nitrobenzene	–	negative
p-Chloronitrobenzene	–	negative
p-Dichlorobenzene	–	negative
1,2,4-Trichlorobenzene	–	negative
1,2,4,5-Tetrachlorobenzene	–	negative
Hexachlorobenzene	–	negative

Guinea pigs were sensitized by repeated intracutaneous injections with solutions of each benzene derivative and were tested 2 wk later by an intracutaneous injection at the same dose used for sensitization.
Source: From Landsteiner and Jacobs (1936).

Control individuals did show some reactions, but to a larger dose of tuberculin. The test was later modified by Mantoux (1910), where the material to be tested was introduced by an intradermal, instead of a subcutaneous, injection. The introduction of the Mantoux test made possible the quantitative study of conditions under which experimental sensitization can be produced. Guinea pigs and rabbits proved to be particularly suitable experimental animals for these studies. In addition, the use of adjuvant, such as paraffin oil or wax, facilitates sensitization (Coulaud, 1935; Freund et al., 1938; Freund and McDermott, 1942).

In humans, a positive tuberculin reaction is characterized by a slow start showing a white or pink colored swelling a few hours after injection. The reaction increases in strength in the first 24 hr and attains its peak about 48 hr after injection (Mantoux, 1910). After 24 and 48 hr, macrophages form approximately 15 to 35% of the cell population in the infiltrate; the rest of mononuclear cells are lymphocytes (Turk et al., 1966; Turk, 1975). Polymorphonuclear leucocytes are rarely seen.

Epicutaneous skin tests with simple chemicals such as 1-fluoro-2,4-dinitrobenzene (DNFB) (Eisen et al., 1952), picryl chloride (Chase, 1954) and 2-ethoxymethylene-5-oxazolone (Gell et al., 1946) show reactions that differ somewhat from those caused by intradermal injection of tuberculin. Because of the mode of application, the complex hapten-protein lies not only within the epidermis layers but also is present within the sweat and sebaceous glands (Turk, 1975). As early as 3 hr after testing, the tested areas of the skin become infiltrated with mononuclear cells. The cell infiltration increases and is followed by appearance of intercellular edema at 6 to 12 hr (McCallum, 1957). At 24 hr, the cell population is composed mainly of macrophages (20%) and lymphocytes (80%). At 48 hr after testing, when the reaction is usually at its peak, the proportion of macrophages decreases to 14% of the total cell population (Turk et al., 1966).

Because of similar clinical and histological manifestations, the tuberculin reaction and ACD to simple chemicals have been classified as type IV (delayed hypersensitivity) reactions (Coombs and Gell, 1964).

Transfer of Contact Sensitivity

Delayed hypersensitivity reactions form a class of immunological reactions characterized by a delayed skin test not inhibited by antihistaminic drugs. The reaction persists in the absence of demonstrable antibodies in serum (Chase, 1966; Gell and Hinde, 1951). Most remarkable if the fact that delayed hypersensitivity can be transferred with living leucocytes from a sensitive animal (Table 2) but not with serum (Chase, 1966; Landsteiner and Chase, 1942).

The inability to transfer tuberculin sensitivity with serum was first observed by Zinsser and Mueller (1925) and confirmed by Freund (1926). Although it has been reported that serum can transfer delayed hypersensitivity (Dupuy et al., 1969, 1970a,b; Dupuy and Good, 1970, 1971; Perey et al., 1970), these results have been questioned by others (Indgin and Inderbitzin, 1971; Richardson and Paterson, 1973). Serum transfer appears to transmit immediate rather than delayed sensitivity (Richardson and Paterson, 1973). Successful passive transfer in the guinea pig has been reported using peritoneal exudate (Chase, 1945; Kantor and Dixon, 1972; Landsteiner and Chase, 1942),

Table 2 Comparison of the Ability of Living and Killed Leukocytes to Transfer Picryl Chloride Sensitivity

Cell source	Number of living cells transferred[a]	Intensity of the skin reaction	Frozen and thawed (+ DNase)[b]	Sonicated[c]
Peritoneal exudates	2.5×10^4	+++++	$3X$[d]	0.68X
Lymph nodes				
Pool 1	9.5×10^8	++++	3.4X	1X
Pool 2	7.6×10^5	++++	1.3X	2X
Spleens			3.3X	2.5X
Pool 1	5.6×10^8	+++	3.2X	1X
Pool 2	7.1×10^8	+++	1.3X	2X
			2.7X	2.8X
Results of transfer of disrupted cells			0/7	0/9

[a]Cells were taken from guinea pigs sensitized chiefly to picryl and chloride by the "combination" method. Animals were injected at five sites with 0.2 ml each of a suspension of picrylated guinea pig erythrocyte stromata (10 mg) and 0.5 mg of killed *Mycobacterium tuberculosis*. Initial injections were followed by treatment of the animals with picryl chloride (1%) in olive oil.

[b]Freezings and thawings, in quite varied menstrua, were done in succession five to eight times.

[c]Sonication was conducted in polypropylene tubes within the cooled chamber of a 9-kv Raytheon oscillator until cells were disrupted as seen by phase-contrast microscopy.

[d]Multiples of living control cells.

Animals were skin tested with 1% picryl chloride in olive oil, 1 to 2 days after injection of cells.

Source: From Chase (1966).

thymus cells (Haxthausen, 1947, 1951), spleen cells (Kirchheimer and Weiser, 1947), and lymph node cells (Bauer and Stone, 1961).

Additional evidence that the delayed reaction is a cellular rather than a humoral response comes from the findings that agammaglobulinemic patients can show delayed hypersensitivity (Good et al., 1957), that antilymphocyte antisera prevent sensitization (Inderbitzin, 1956; Waskman and Arbouys, 1962), and that delayed hypersensitive response can be impaired by immune cell deficiencies (Chilgren et al., 1967; Cooper et al., 1973; Valdimarsson et al., 1973).

Transfer of bacterial allergy in man can be accomplished reproducibly (Lawrence, 1949; 1972-1973), but it appears to be more difficult to transfer sensitivity to chemical agents (Baer and Sulzberger, 1952; Baer et al., 1952; Harber and Baer, 1961; Haxthausen, 1953). Positive results have been reported (Epstein and Kligman, 1957; Good et al., 1957), although they have not been confirmed. It is difficult to know whether a true passive transfer of delayed hypersensitivity to chemicals has been demonstrated in humans. Further work is required to determine if a specific increase in skin reactivity has been induced by injection of cells or by boosting of an already existing low sensitivity.

In guinea pigs, the fate of the injected sensitized cells has been investigated using cells labeled with tritium or ^{32}P. It was shown (Hamilton and Chase, 1962; Kay and Rieke, 1963; McCluskey et al., 1963; Najarian and Feldman, 1961; Turk, 1962; Turk and Oort, 1963) that after 24 hr, 40 to 50% of the cells are found in the liver while about 2% remain in the circulation. Labeled cells take part in delayed hypersensitivity as observed in autoradiographies of lesions in the subepidermal dermis. In addition, it was found that 90% or more of the cells infiltrating the lesion after passive transfer were of recipient origin; donor cells did not appear to make any significant contribution to the cellular infiltrate.

Transfer of bacterial sensitivity has been studied extensively. The pioneering work of Lawrence showed that not only viable leucocytes could transfer sensitivity (Lawrence, 1949) but also that extracts prepared from these cells were as effective (Lawrence, 1955). The latter observation led to the concept of the transfer factor (Lawrence, 1955). Transfer factor is prepared by osmotic lysis of sensitive leucocytes or by freezing and thawing the cells. Successful and best reproducible transfers of cutaneous delayed-type hypersensitivity are observed when cells from a donor showing a strong positive cutaneous reaction are used. In addition, it has been shown that a minimum number of sensitized leucocytes (85 to 170 $\times$ 10^6 cells) must be used for systemic transfer of bacterial allergy (Lawrence, 1955). Transfer factor has been used to transfer positively sensitivity to tuberculin, streptococcal M substance, diphtheria toxoid, and coccidioidin (reviewed by Lawrence, 1972-1973).

Transfer factor is a specific substance that can be produced in vitro by incubating leucocytes with antigen (Lawrence, 1969). The substance is a water-soluble, dialyzable, low-molecular-weight ($<$10,000) polypeptide-polynucleotide complex that is stable to lyophilization. Purification of transfer factor by dialysis and gel filtration has established that the substance is highly potent in selectively transferring bacterial cutaneous sensitivity without production of antibodies in humans or in experimental animals. The structure of transfer factor remains to be established and represents an interesting challenge for a substance that may find extensive application in the therapy of diseases either arising from or resulting in defects of cellular immunity (Lawrence, 1972-1973).

Nature of the Cells Implicated
in Delayed Hypersensitivity and in ACD

Lymphocytes are the specific cells of the immune system. Evidence has accumulated to indicate that two different populations of lymphocytes are responsible for immune responsiveness (Ford, 1973; Katz and Benacerraf, 1972; Miller and Mitchell, 1968; Raff, 1973; Roitt et al., 1969). Lymphoid cells have been classified as thymus-dependent (T cells) or thymus-independent (B or bursa-equivalent) cells.

In the embryo, lymphoid stem cells originate in blood islets in the yolk sac and, subsequently, in the fetal liver and bone marrow. Progeny of the bone marrow stem cells migrate either through a specific organ in birds, called the bursa of Fabricius, or through the thymus. In all other species, cells migrate through the thymus or through the bursa-equivalent regions (Cooper et al., 1967, 1968; Good et al., 1966). In man, the nature of bursa-equivalent regions remains unknown. Bone marrow itself (Abdou and Abdou, 1972), the gastrointestinal lymphoid organs (Archer et al., 1963; Cooper et al., 1966; Perey et al., 1968; Peterson et al., 1965), or the hemopoietic tissues (Abdou and Richter, 1970; Brahim and Osmond, 1970; Nossal and Pike, 1973) have been suggested as possible bursa equivalents.

Lymphoid organs, such as the thymus and the bursa of Fabricius (or its equivalent), provide a microenvironment necessary for the maturation of lymphocytes. It is now well established that several hormones participate in this process. The best characterized of these hormones are: thymosin α_1 (Goldstein et al., 1977; Low and Goldstein, 1979), thymopoietin I and II (Goldstein, 1974; Schlesinger and Goldstein, 1975), ubiquitin (Schlesinger et al., 1975), and the *facteur thymique sérique* (Bach et al., 1977; Pleau et al., 1977). Other hormones or factors have been shown to exist, but their chemical structure has not been reported. Among these factors are: (1) the thymic humoral factor (Trainin et al., 1975a,b), (2) a factor possessing thymic hormone-like activity in human blood identified as prealbumin (White and Burton, 1979), and (3) bursopoietin, a lymphocyte-differentiating hormone of the bursa of Fabricius (Brand et al., 1976). A review on the properties of these hormones and factors has appeared (Bach and Carnaud, 1976).

Immunocompetent B and T cells possess characteristic properties and their functions in immune responses are different. B cells are the precursors of antibody-secreting plasma cells (Mitchell and Miller, 1968; Nossal et al., 1968), whereas T cells cooperate in the stimulation or suppression of B-cell activity (Claman and Chaperon, 1969; Katz and Benacerraf, 1972; Miller and Mitchell, 1969; Mitchison et al., 1970; Raff, 1970a,b; Raff and Wortis, 1970; Taylor, 1969) and are also responsible for cellular immunity, which encompasses delayed hypersensitivity (Gell and Benacerraf, 1961; Gell and Silverstein, 1962), protection against viral, fungal, and bacterial pathogens (Blanden, 1974), immunological surveillance against oncogenesis (Cerottini and Brunner, 1974; Henney, 1973), transplantation immunity (Blomgren et al., 1970; Cerottini et al., 1970; Sprent and Miller 1972a,b), recognition of the carrier in allergies to chemicals (Mitchison, 1971a,b; Rubin et al., 1973), and the capacities to give mixed lymphocyte reactions (Kisken and Swenson, 1969; Knight et al., 1973; Wilson et al., 1967).

The two cell populations are further differentiated by surface properties of their plasma membranes. Bone marrow-derived cells (B-cells) can be identified by the presence of easily detectable immunoglobulins (Raff, 1970b; Uhr and Vitetta, 1973; Unanue et al., 1973; Wigzell and Andersson, 1969) on their surfaces. Most B cells also possess a receptor for antigen-antibody-complement complexes (Bianco et al., 1970; Eden et al., 1971; Lay and Nussenzweig, 1968; Shevach et al., 1973; Uhr and Phillips, 1966) and a receptor for the F_c portion of immunoglobulin G (Basten et al., 1972a,b; Dickler and Kunkel, 1972; Paraskevas et al., 1972). Furthermore, it has been shown that B lymphocytes adhere to anti-immunoglobulin antibody coated solid surfaces (Walters and Wigzell, 1970; Wigzell and Andersson, 1969) and that antigen absorption can be prevented by anti-immunoglobulin reagents (Ada et al., 1970). B cells also possess alloantigenic surface markers. In the mouse, these lymphocytes carry the Ly antigen system (Ly-4, Ly-6, Ly-7, Lyb-8) (Snell et al., 1973).

T cells carry specific alloantigenic, serologically defined, surface markers. In mice, T lymphocytes possess the theta iso-antigen (Thy-1.1, Thy-1.2) (Raff, 1969; Raff and Wortis, 1970; Schlesinger and Yron, 1969; Schlesinger, 1970) and the TL (Boyse and Old, 1969), Ly-1 (Itakura et al., 1972), Ly-2 (Itakura et al., 1972), and Ly-3 (Shigeno et al., 1968) antigens. In man, T cells can form rosettes with sheep red blood cells (Bach et al., 1970; Bach, 1973; Greaves and Möller, 1970a,b) and with haptenated red blood cells (Möller et al., 1971; Möller and Mäkelä, 1972). The nature of the T-cell receptor for antigens remains, however, controversial. There have been reports suggesting an immunoglobulin-like nature for that receptor (Greaves, 1970; Marchalonis, 1975; Marchalonis et al., 1978; Paul, 1973).

The nature, distribution, and properties of lymphocyte plasma membrane markers have been extensively discussed by Katz (1977).

The stimulation of antibody-forming cells, in response to antigens, requires collaboration between T cells and B cells (Cheers et al., 1971; Claman and Chaperon, 1969; Davies, 1969; Miller and Mitchell, 1968, 1969; Miller, 1971; Miller et al., 1971; Mitchell, G.F., et al., 1971; Mitchison et al., 1970; Mitchison, 1971a,b; Moorhead et al., 1973; Paul et al., 1970; Raff, 1970a; Taylor, 1969). Cellular collaboration (T-B cells) is also essential for production of antihapten (DNP) antibodies (Janeway, 1975a,b) and for the "carrier effect" phenomenon (Mitchison, 1971a,b). For primary and secondary in vitro responses to heterologous erythrocytes or to antigens, an additional requirement for macrophages or other phagocytic cells is essential (Cline and Sweet, 1968; Feldman and Palmer, 1971; Gordon, 1968; Hersh and Harris, 1968; Moorhead et al., 1973; Oppenheim et al., 1968; Pierce et al., 1974; Shortman et al., 1970; Shortman and Palmer, 1971; Watson et al., 1974).

In ACD to simple chemiclas, other types of cells may also be implicated. Recent findings have shown that in actively sensitized (DNCB) patients or guinea pigs, Langerhans cells are frequently found apposed by mononuclear cells, and this observation has led to the postulate that Langerhans cells play an important role in the cutaneous reaction to simple chemicals (Silberberg et al., 1974a,b, 1975, 1976). Apposition at the sites of contact allergic reactions can occur as early as 3 to 5 hr after challenge and is seen in active sensitization in man and in the guinea pig as well as in passive sensitization in guinea pigs (Silberberg et al., 1976). Apposition is not seen in contact primary irritant reactions (Silberberg, 1971). Close examination by electron microscopy of the reaction sites reveals that Langerhans cells apposed to mononuclear cells show morphologic changes suggestive of cellular activity. These changes consist of prominent channels of endoplasmic reticulum and of lysosomes. These observations, together with the suggestion that Langerhans cells are epidermal macrophages (Hashimoto, 1971) and that they occur in the lymph nodes and the thymus, suggest that these cells may be involved not only in contact allergic reactions but also in other immunologic reactions, particularly in cell-mediated reactions in the skin.

Induction and Elicitation of the Immune Response in ACD

The process of sensitization to contact allergens may be divided into two mains phases: induction and elicitation of the response (Polak, 1977, 1980). The inductive phase can be further subdivided into three temporally separated events.

1. Formation of hapten-protein conjugate,
2. Recognition of the conjugate by cells of the immune system, and
3. Proliferation and dissemination of sensitized lymphocytes endowed with specific effector and memory properties.

The phase of elicitation of the immune response takes place after repeated contact of the same antigen (conjugate) with effector cells. These repeated challenges result in the production of a local inflammatory reaction.

The Inductive Phase

The first step of the inductive phase in ACD consists of the formation of hapten conjugates with skin or serum proteins or with circulating cells (further discussed in Chap 5). Part of the hapten remains bound to protein components of the skin, whereas the rest is carried bound to proteins into the lymphatic vessel of the draining lymph node (McFarlin and Balfour, 1973; Hall and Smith, 1971) or the blood stream (in bound or free form). Unconjugated hapten is eliminated via urine and feces (Godfrey et al., 1971).

The second step consists of antigen recognition by antigen-inexperienced lymphoctyes. The process of recognition (sensitization) appears to take place at the level of the skin. Evidence in support of this concept has come from the findings that the hapten must persist in the skin for a certain length of time. For instance, in the guinea pig, excision of the site of hapten application up to 8 hr after application prevents sensitization (Frey and Wenk, 1957; Macher and Chase, 1969; Turk and Stone, 1963). Cells, after being stimulated, travel to the draining lymph node where they proliferate and differentiate. The importance of this mechanism was demonstrated by the classical work of Frey and Wenk (1957). Skin islands from guinea pigs' flanks were cut out and isolated from surrounding skin and underlying tissues, leaving intact blood and lymphatic vessels, nerves, and skin syncytium. The authors were able to show that hypersensitivity was induced only when lymphatic vessels were left intact. Interruption of blood flow or nerve or skin connections had no influence.

Proliferation of hapten-sensitive lymphocytes occurs in the paracortical area of the lymph node (Macher, 1962a,b,c; Macher and Chase, 1969; Turk and Oort, 1970). These small lymphocytes transform into immunoblasts, which divide and give rise to small lymphocytes (Turk and Stone, 1963) with effector and memory properties. The lymphocytes that leave the draining lymph node comprise mainly two major populations: (1) the memory lymphocyte population, which circulates between the thymus-dependent areas of the lymph nodes, the spleen, and the lymphatic vessels, and (2) the effector lymphocytes, which circulate in the peripheral blood. These cells are able to induce an inflammatory skin reaction but cannot proliferate and differentiate.

The Eliciting Phase

The eliciting phase can be demonstrated in sensitive patients or experimental animals by topical or subcutaneous application of the hapten. The hapten reacts with carrier proteins, forming a conjugate that is identical or resembles (see Chap. 7 for a discussion of cross-reactivity) the one to which cells are sensitive. The result is an inflammatory reaction that peaks 24 to 48 hr after challenge. Phagocytic cells (macrophages, Langerhans cells) are probably involved in the "presentation" or recognition of the hapten-protein conjugate by sensitive (effector) lymphocytes.

2

In Vitro Studies of Delayed Hypersensitivity

The complex phenomenon of delayed hypersensitivity can be studied in vitro.
Various experimental tests have been shown to correlate with delayed hypersensitivity, among which are the lymphocyte transformation test (Cowling et
al., 1963; Ling and Kay, 1975; Pearmain et al., 1963) and the inhibition of
macrophage migration from capillary tubes (Bloom and Bennett, 1966; David,
1966; David and David, 1972; George and Vaughan, 1962; Melnick, 1971).

The Lymphocyte Transformation Test

Small lymphocytes can be induced to transform in vitro into large blast-like
cells, which are able to synthesize DNA and to divide. Such stimulation can
be triggered by various lectins (Hungerford et al., 1959; Lis and Sharon,
1973; Nowell, 1960; Sharon and Lis, 1972), specific immune antigens (Cowling et al., 1963; Heilman and McFarland, 1966a,b; Hirschhorn et al., 1964;
McFarland and Heilman, 1966; Pearmain et al., 1963; Sarkany and Caron,
1966), antileukocytes antisera (Grasbeck et al., 1964), histocompatability
antigens (Bain et al., 1964), myeloma proteins (Leon and Takahashi, 1970),
antiallotypicglobulin antisera (Sell and Gell, 1965), enzymes (Novogrodsky
and Katchalsky, 1973), drugs (Mathews et al., 1972; Zweiman and Silberberg,
1971), haptens conjugated to a carrier (Dupuis, 1979; Milner, 1970, 1971,
1974), periodate (Novogrodsky and Katchalsky, 1971), and a calcium ionophore (Green et al., 1976).

The degree of lymphocyte transformation is usually assayed by enumera-

Table 1 In Vitro [^{3}H] Thymidine Incorporation (cpm) by Lymphocytes From Humans Sensitized to 2,4-Dinitro-1-fluorobenzene and Stimulated by 2,4-Dinitrophenyl Skin Protein Conjugates

	Subjects					
Stimulating agent[a]	B.M.	W.S.	R.S.	C.K.	E.R.	T.G.
SP (50 μg)	348	743	830	479	451	188
DNP-SP (50 μg)	1,945	4,421	5,315	2,680	1,100	1,744
None	232	321	1,157	335	362	138
Skin test	4+	4+	4+	4+	4+	4+
Ratio (DND-SP/SP)	5.6	6.0	6.4	5.6	2.4	9.3
PWM	33,463	25,055	89,650	43,568	33,524	66,402

[a]Abbreviations: SP, skin proteins; DNP-SP, dinitrophenyl skin proteins; PWM, pokeweed mitogen; cpm, counts per minute.

Skin proteins were prepared by freezing and thawing fresh tissue in Tris-HCl buffer (pH, 8.4). DNP-SP conjugates were prepared by reacting 1-fluoro-2,4-dinitrobenzene (DNFB) with skin extracts. Lymphocytes obtained by venipuncture were incubated (1 $\times$ 10^6 cells/ml) in Waymouth's medium for 5 days. Cells were harvested, acid treated, and the amount of [^{3}H] thymidine incorporated was determined.

Subjects have been experimentally sensitized to DNFB.

Source: From Milner (1974). © 1974 The Williams & Wilkins Co., Baltimore.

Table 2 Characteristics of Some Lymphokines

Lymphokines	Properties
Macrophage migration inhibition factor (MIF)	inhibits macrophage movement in vitro
Leukotactic factor (LF)	attracts leucocytes in vitro
Skin reactive factor (SRF)	produces induration, erythema, and mononuclear cell infiltration after intradermal injection
Lymphotoxin (LT)	a cytotoxin produced in vitro that does not act on lymphocytes
Macrophage aggregation factor (MAF)	agglutinates macrophages in vitro
Mitogenic factor	induces DNA synthesis in lymphocytes in vitro
Lymph node permeability factor	increases vascular permeability
Interferon	prevents viral replication in target cells

tion of lymphoblasts, measuring increases in DNA content, or measuring the incorporation of precursors in proteins or nucleic acids (Bloom, 1971; Bloom and Glade, 1971) (Table 1).

Lymphocytes in culture produce, under stimulation, a number of factors collectively referred to as lymphokines (Dumonde et al., 1969). The lymphokines include: a macrophage migration inhibition factor (MIF) (Bloom and Bennett, 1966; David, 1966; Remold et al., 1970), a leukotactic factor (LF) (Ward et al., 1970), a skin reactive factor (SRF) (Bennett and Bloom, 1968), lymphotoxins (LTs) (Granger and Williams, 1968; Kolb and Granger, 1968), a macrophage aggregation factor (MAF) (Gotoff and Vizral, 1972; Nathan et al., 1971), a mitogenic factor (Gordon and MacLean, 1965; Kasakura and Lowenstein, 1965), a lymph node permeability factor (Willoughby et al., 1962), and a factor possessing interferon-like activity (Green et al., 1969) (Table 2).

The Macrophage Migration Inhibition Test

This test is based upon the observation that peritoneal exudate cells from guinea pigs that exhibit strong in vivo response to an antigen are inhibited from migrating out of capillary tubes in the presence of that antigen. Cells from nonsensitive animals migrate normally (George and Vaughan, 1962). The test can be used as the direct (David and David, 1971), semidirect (Rosenstreich et al., 1971; Rosenstreich and Rosenthal, 1974), and indirect methods (Bloom and Bennett, 1971). In the semidirect method, a mixed cell population containing approximately 10% lymphocytes from a hypersensitive animal and 90% peritoneal exudate from a nonimmune animal are assayed in the presence of the antigen used for immunization. In the indirect method, supernatants obtained after incubation of sensitive lymphocytes with and without specific antigen are added to peritoneal exudate cells from nonsensitive naimals. Assays are performed in the presence of antigen and only supernatants containing MIF show a positive response (Fig. 1).

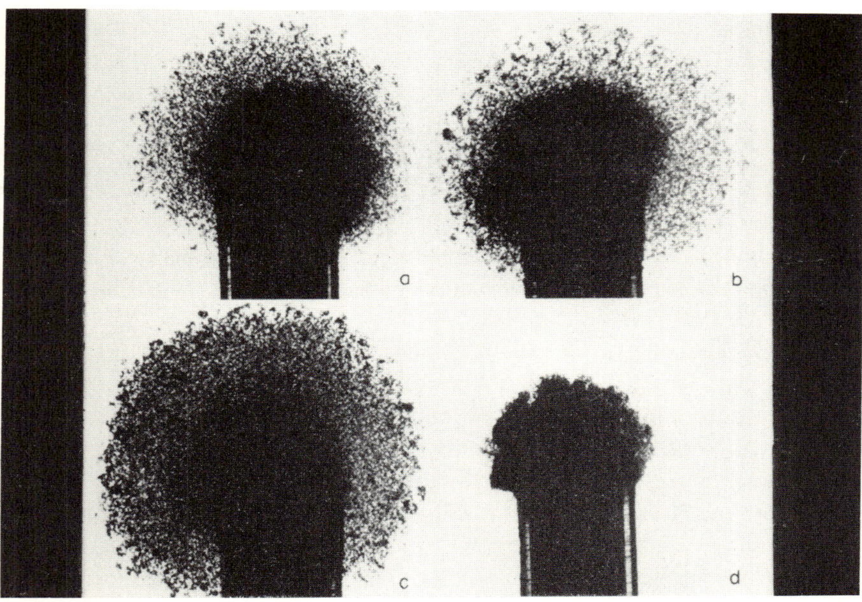

Figure 1 Specific inhibition of migration of periteneal exudate cells from 2,4-dinitrochlorobenzene (DNCB) sensitized guinea pigs with DNP-serum conjugate. The conjugate was prepared by reaction of DNCB with serum, in sodium carbonate buffer. (*a*) Normal cells in control media, (*b*) normal cells with DNP-serum conjugate, (*c*) sensitized cells in control media, (*d*) sensitized cells incubated in the presence of DNP-serum conjugate. Magnification is 15X. (From Friend and Lane, 1973).

The phenomenon can be observed using cells sensitive to paraphenylene-diamine (PPD) (Bloom and Bennett, 1966; David et al., 1964a,b), hapten-protein conjugates (David et al., 1964c; Friend and Lane, 1973; Herman and Sams, 1971), keyhole limpet hemocyanin (Curtis and Hersh, 1973), transplantation antigens (Malmgren et al., 1969; Mills, 1966), metal salts (Hutchison et al., 1972; Mirza et al., 1974; Polak and Frey, 1973; Thulin and Zacharinae, 1972), synthetic polypeptides (David and Schlossman, 1968), carbohydrates (God-frey et al., 1969), viruses (Feinstone et al., 1969), antibiotics (Nordqvist and Rorsman, 1967), tumor antigens (Kronman et al., 1969), and to pathogenic organisms (Biberfeld, 1973; Boros et al., 1973).

Correlation of In Vitro Tests with Delayed Hypersensitivity

Lymphocyte transformation and macrophage migration inhibition in the presence of antigens have been correlated to cell-mediated immune reactions in vivo (Astor et al., 1973; Biberfeld, 1973; Bloom and Bennett, 1966, 1969, 1970; Bloom et al., 1969; Bloom and Jimenez, 1970; Bloom, 1971; Borel and David, 1970; Boros et al., 1973, David et al., 1964c; Geczy and Baumgarten, 1970; Hanna et al., 1973; Kronman et al., 1969; Mills, 1966; Milner, 1971, 1972; Oppenheim, 1968; Polak and Frey, 1973). The correlation has been established from the findings that these two tests are antigen specific, positive only in sensitized animals, positive in sensitized animals without detectable circulating antibodies, negative in animals possessing only circulating antibodies, and negative in animals made tolerant to the specific antigen. The tests show also carrier specificity.

In some circumstances, however, the lymphocyte transformation test and macrophage migration inhibition test may be discordant, suggesting that different lymphocyte populations are involved (Rocklin et al., 1970; Rocklin, 1973).

3

In Vivo Studies of
Delayed Hypersensitivity

The identification of an allergen (hapten) responsible for a recurring eczema is done by testing. The most common procedure in man is the *challenge test*: the substance suspected to be the causative agent is tested at subtoxic concentrations. This procedure applies to naturally sensitized people. Sensitization is sometimes voluntarily induced in humans. Since this may lead to permanent sensitivity to the sensitizer(s) (and possible cross-reactivity to other haptens), controversial opinions exist about the ethics of the procedure; animal models are therefore preferred.

In Vivo Testing in Humans

Experimental Sensitization

In an important series of papers, Kligman (1966a,b,c,d) has described a method of "maximization test" to predict the allergenic potential of chemical substances. In this procedure, the skin is treated with a potent irritant, sodium laurylether (dodecyl) sulfate (SLS), applied as an occlusive patch for 24 hr. The irritating agent is then removed by washings and the test material is applied to the same site for 48 hr. The same sequence of treatment is repeated five times. The challenge test is performed thereafter with the test material and the cutaneous reaction is read at 24 and at 48 hr.

This "maximization test" procedure has allowed Kligman to classify chemical substances into five categories, graded 1 to 5, according to the cutaneous

Table 1 Grading of Various Chemical Substances as to Their Ability to Produce Cutaneous Reactions in Humans Tested by the "Maximization Test" Procedure

Number of sensitized individuals	Classification of the cutaneous reaction	Grade
0 to 2/25	weak	1
3 to 7/25	mild	2
8 to 13/25	moderate	3
14 to 20/25	strong	4
21 to 25/25	extreme	5

Twenty five subjects were first submitted to the "maximization test" procedure and then tested with various chemicals including soap, detergents, chemicals, cosmetics, drugs, natural compounds, etc. Patch tests were read at 48 hr.
Source: From Kligman (1966d). © 1966 The Williams & Wilkins Co., Baltimore.

reactions observed with the 25 patients tested (Kligman, 1966d). Kligman's classification is summarized in Table 1.

The conditions for the "maximization test" have been recently modified from the point of view of irritant concentration and procedure of maximization (Kligman and Eptein, 1975). Other methods are also used (Marzulli and Maibach, 1976). They are, however, modifications of older ones.

The various methods used in experimental sensitization in humans provide results that may be used as a guide concerning the allergenic potency of chemical substances. The predictive value of these methods must not, however, be taken too rigidly. In the case of the "maximization test," Kligman' view is that the test is not "prophetic" but that its objective is "to establish whether specified substances have allergenic potentialities and to what degree" (Kligman, 1966d).

Table 2 summarizes the allergenic potentiality of chemicals tested according to Kligman's procedure.

Challenge Tests

The aim of the test is to provoke a "minieczema" reminiscent of the real one. The first use of the patch test was described by Jadassohn (1895, 1896). To-

day, the open cutaneous technique is rarely used. The procedure has been
replaced by the occlusive patch test. There is, however, a lack of standardized
conditions—for instance, the brand of adhesive tape and the vehicle and concentrations of the testing substance vary from one clinic (or dermatologist's
office) to another. Some attempts at standardization have been put forward. Standard kits of allergens for patch testing are commercially avail-
able. Unfortunately, the concentration of each individual sample in the
kit varies greatly, even as much as 15-fold on a molar basis (Benezra et al.,
1978).

The most common procedure for patch testing is to deposit the hapten
in solution, emulsion, or dispersion in a solvent or petrolatum onto a filter
paper (or a linen), which is then fixed on the patient's back (or, less frequently, on the forearm) and covered with an adhesive tape. Readings are
made 24 and 48 hr later, and the intensity of the cutaneous reaction is
graded with a plus (+) sign. The convention for the number of (+) signs
is not universally accepted. The one used by the international Contact
Dermatitis Research Group (ICDRG) is as follows:

0   No reaction

?+   Doubtful reaction

+   Weak (nonvesicular) reaction

++   Strong (edematous and vesicular) reaction

+++   Extreme reaction

IR   Irritant

Control patch tests (on nonsensitive patients) should always be performed
to ensure that, at the concentration tested, the substance is not an irritant.
Other test procedures such as intradermal testing and patch testing on
mucous membranes are sometimes used (Hjorth and Fregert, 1979).

Some substances are photoactive; they are allergenic only after activation by light. Testing in this case requires a special technique—the photo
patch testing. Here, the substance is deposited on the skin and the site is
irradiated with ultraviolet light. Nonirradiated sites with the same substance
serve as controls.

A summary of the various patch-test procedures has appeared (Hjorth
and Fregert, 1979).

Table 2 Allergenic Potentialities of Various Chemicals Determined by the "Maximization Test" Procedure

Grade	Classification of the cutaneous reaction	Chemical substances tested			
		Topical agents	Antimicrobial agents	Industrial contactants	Systemic drugs
1	weak	SLS petrolatum lanolin Tween 80 Xylocaine resorcinol	griseofulvin Bacitracin phenol Chloromycetin sulfathiazole hexachlorophene bithionol Vioform	benzene xylene pyridine dimethylsulfoxide hexane	thiabendazole testosterone hydrocortisone 8-methoxypsoralene
2	mild	procaine HCl benzocaine	sulfonilamide tetramethylthiuram- disulfide Neomycin	anilide	

3	moderate	brutyne sulfate Nupercaine	kanamycin procaine penicillin ammoniated mercury	mercapto- benzothiazole nickel sulfate chromium oxide chromium sulfate	Phenergan Furacin
4	strong		penicillin G streptomycin Furacin formalin	cobaltous sulfate gold chloride turpentine butyl diglycyl ether beryllium sulfate	chlorpromazin Atabrin

5	extreme	hydroquinone
		   monobenzylether
		PPD
			mercuric chloride
			tetrachlorosalicyl-
			   anilide
				potassium dichromate
				diethylenetriamine
				diethyl fumarate
				malathion
				glyoxal
				hydrazine
				epoxy resin
					Apressoline
					BAL

Source: From Kligman (1966d). © 1966 The Williams & Wilkins Co., Baltimore.

In Vivo Testing of Animals

Sensitization

Several animals have been used as models for studying allergic contact dermatitis (ACD): guinea pigs (Coulaud, 1935; Dienes, 1928; Saentz, 1938), monkeys (Strauss, 1937), rabbits (Frey and Geleick, 1959), pigs (McFarlin and Balfour, 1973), sheep (Hall and Smith, 1971), mice (Asherson and Ptak, 1968), and dogs (Nobréus et al., 1974; Rostenberg and Haeberlin, 1950). Reviews of contact hypersensitivity in experimental animals have appeared (Maibach, 1975; Parker and Turk, 1974; Stork, 1962).

Several methods of sensitization in experimental animals exist and they have been critically reviewed by Klecak (1977; Klecak et al. 1977). The most important ones include:

1. Epicutaneous methods (Bühler's test and open epicutaneous test),
2. Intradermal techniques (Draize's test, complete Freund's adjuvant [CFA] test),
3. Method using both application routes (split adjuvant technique and guinea pig maximization test).

These methods will be reviewed briefly here. Additional details can be found in Klecak's review (1977).

Draize's Method (Draize, 1955)

Induction of contact sensitivity is made by 10 intradermal injections (one every other day) of the hapten in aqueous sodium chloride, paraffin, or polyethyleneglycol. Challenge is performed 2 weeks after the last injection by intradermally injecting the same solution (or emulsion), and the response is evaluated.

Freund's Complete Adjuvant Method (Klecak et al., 1977)

CFA (killed *Mycobacterium* suspended in mineral oil) enhances sensitization. The induction period includes five intradermal injections of the hapten in CFA, every other day. Two weeks after the last injection, a solution of the hapten is applied epicutaneously onto the shaved flank of the animal. The reaction is evaluated at 24 and at 48 hr.

The Bühler Test (Bühler and Griffith, 1975)

The procedure consists in an occlusive patch test of the hapten in the appropriate vehicle, for a duration of 6 hr. The process is repeated 1 week and then

2 weeks later. Challenge is also performed with an occlusive patch test. The reaction is evaluated at 24, 48, and 72 hr.

The Open Epicutaneous Test (Klecak, 1977, Klecak et al., 1977)

The induction consists of the daily application of the hapten, in a suitable vehicle, for a period of 2 to 3 weeks until a strong positive reaction occurs. Challenge is performed by open epicutaneous testing, 2 weeks after the last application of hapten.

The Guinea Pig Maximization Test (Magnusson and Kligman, 1969, 1970)

The first day, six intradermal injections of the hapten are done. Two of these injections comprise the hapten in a suitable vehicle, two comprise CFA alone, and two comprise the hapten in the vehicle plus CFA. Seven days later, a petrolatum dispersion of the hapten is applied epicutaneously (occlusive patch test) on the three previously injected areas. After 48 hr, the adhesive tape is removed. Challenge is performed 12 days later (by occlusive patches), and the reaction is read at 3 hr and 24 hr.

The Split Adjuvant Technique (Maguire, 1973)

This method combines the occlusive tests and the intradermal injections of CFA plus hapten. Challenge is effected (occlusive test) 3 weeks after the first day of induction.

The Optimization Method (Maurer et al., 1975)

Maurer's method combines intradermal injections of the hapten alone (first week) with injection of a suspension of the hapten in CFA (second and third week). Challenge (intradermal test) is done 4 weeks after the first injection. Two weeks after the intradermal challenge, an open epicutaneous test is done. The method seems appropriate for predictive evaluation of sensitizing power for strong (Maurer et al., 1978) and for weak (Maurer et al., 1979) allergens.

In addition to Klecak's review, a critical evaluation of 11 sensitization techniques in experimental animals has appeared (Fahr et al., 1976).

Challenge Tests

Challenge tests have been reviewed in a previous section of this chapter. An example of sensitization and testing of α-methylene-γ-butyrolactones is shown in Table 3. Guinea pigs were sensitized to two naturally occurring α-methylene sesquiterpene lactones, alantolactone, and isoalantolactone. The animals were challenged with natural and synthetic lactones (Stampf et al., 1978). Structures of the lactones tested appear in Figure 1.

Table 3 Results of Epicutaneous Tests in Guinea Pigs Sensitized to Alantolactone and Isoalantolactone

Animals sensitized to	Challenged with	Concentration of test (% w/v) substance	Epicutaneous test[a]				Average[b]	
			3+	2+	+	0	experimental animals	control
Alantolactone	alantolactone (N)[c]	0.1	2	4	3	1	1.7	0
	isoalantolactone (N)	0.1	0	3	6	1	0.7	0
	norbornane lactone (S)	0.1	0	0	2	8	0.2	0
	spirolactone (S)	0.1	0	0	9	1	0.9	0
	frullanolide (N)	0.1	0	4	5	1	1.3	0
	laurenobiolide (N)	0.1	0	1	6	3	0.8	0
	costunolide (N)	0.1	0	0	1	9	0.1	0
	α-methylene-γ butyro-lactone (S)	0.1	0	0	0	10	0	0

Isoalantolactone	isoalantolactone (N)	0.1	3	1	3	0	2.0	0
	alantolactone (N)	0.1	0	3	4	0	1.4	0
	norbornane lactone (S)	0.1	0	0	2	5	0.3	0
	spirolactone (S)	0.1	0	2	4	1	1.1	0
	frullanolide (N)	0.1	0	2	4	1	1.1	0
	laurenobiolide (N)	0.1	0	0	1	6	0.14	0
	costunolide (N)	0.1	0	0	2	0	1.0	0
	α-methylene-γ butyro-lactone (S)	0.1	0	0	0	7	0	0

Animals were sensitized by Magnusson and Kligman's "maximization test" method with 1% solution of alantolactone or isoalantolactone in 1% (w/v) solution of olive oil-acetone (4:1). Test substances were in olive oil-acetone (1:9). Epicutaneous reactions were graded as follows: 3+ = intense erythema, infiltration, and exudation; 2+ = distinct confluent erythema and infiltration; + = distinct erythema; 0 = no reaction.

[a]Number of animals with 0 (n), + (z), 2+ (y), and 3+ (x) skin test intensities.

[b]Averages were calculated by assigning values of 3 for a +++ cutaneous reaction, 2 for ++, and 1 for + and applying the following equation: $3x + 2y + z/x + y + z + n$, respectively. Three control animals were tested with each compound.

[c]N refers to naturally occurring lactones and S refers to synthetic lactones.

Source: Data from Stampf et al. (1978).

64

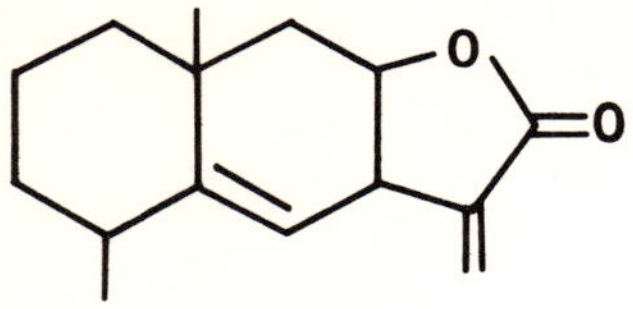

alantolactone

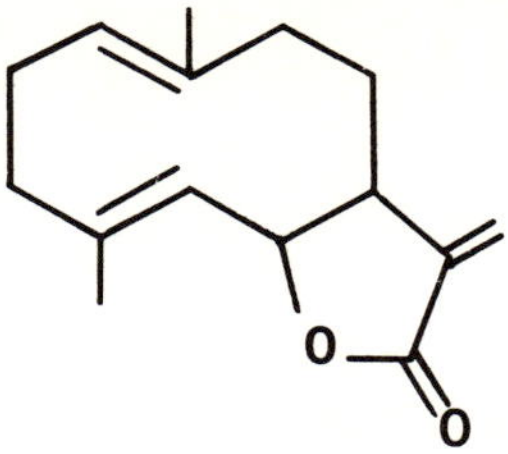

costunolide

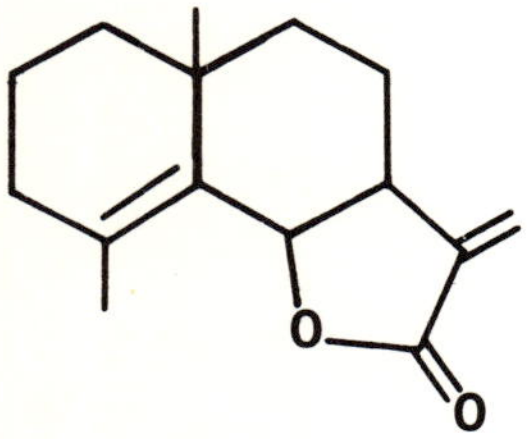

frullanolide

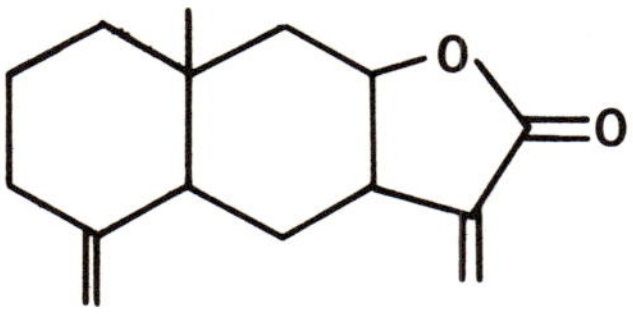

isoalantolactone

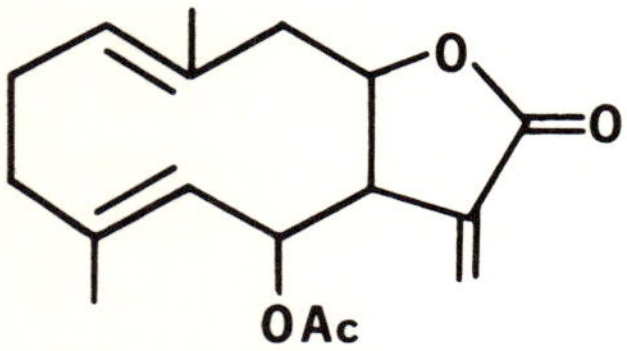

laurenobiolide

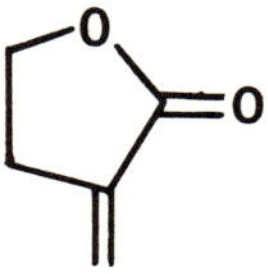

α-methylene-γ-butyrolactone

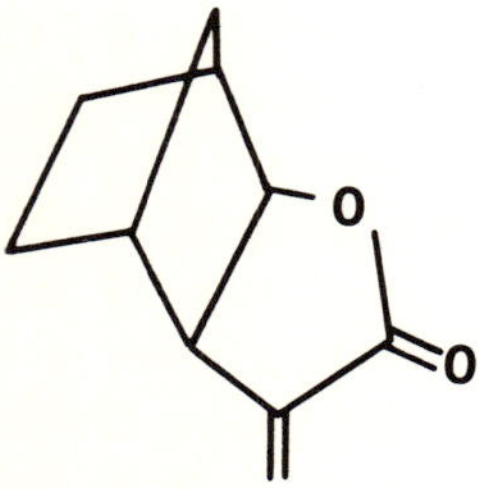

norbornane lactone

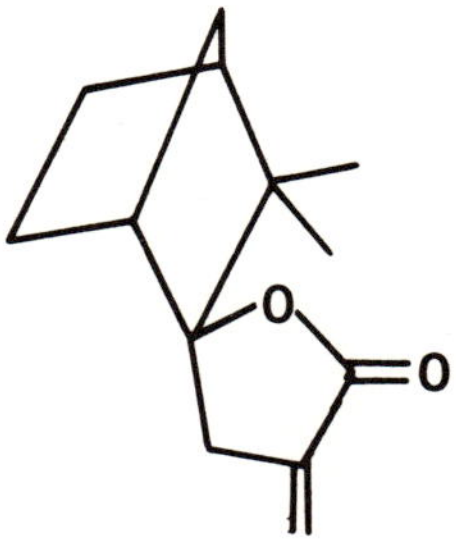

spirolactone

Figure 1 Chemical structures of the various lactones listed in Table 3.

4

The Concept of Carrier in ACD

The concept of carrier in delayed hypersensitivity emerged from work by
Landsteiner's group (Landsteiner and Lampl, 1918; Landsteiner and van der
Scheer, 1928; Landsteiner and Jacobs, 1936; Landsteiner and Chase, 1941),
Eisen (1959), Benacerraf and Gell (1959a,b), and Chase (1966).

Landsteiner and his group observed that guinea pigs injected with hapten-
protein conjugates (picryl bovine gammaglobulin) displayed delayed hypersensitivity to picryl gammaglobulin and to the unconjugated globulin. The
reaction to the unconjugated carrier was greater than that to the picryl-carrier
conjugate. Antibodies could be detected by the Arthus reaction, but only
directed against the conjugate or against the picryl group conjugated to another protein. Delayed hypersensitivity was not detected using the picryl
group attached to another protein but could be observed by using the carrier
alone in the absence of detectable antibodies against it. Eisen's group (Eisen
et al., 1959) attempted to repeat those results, but they reported failure to
induce contact sensitivity to the 2,4-dinitrophenyl (DNP) group using DNP
conjugates. These difficulties since have been overcome, and reproducible results can be obtained with the use of appropriate doses of DNP conjugated to
suitable carriers, such as guinea pig albumin, guinea pig gammaglobulin, or
guinea pig skin proteins (Milner, 1971; Parker et al., 1970; Parker and Turk,
1970; Polak et al., 1974; Salvin and Smith, 1961).

Manifestation of delayed hypersensitivity to hapten-protein conjugates is
greatly influenced by the nature of the carrier. When proteins are used as
carriers, delayed hypersensitivity or recognition by the lymphoid system in

the anamnestic response is directed against the carrier. Polyamino acids, on the other hand, appear not to be as important in the memory response (delayed hypersensitivity) and, in such cases, the hapten is the recognized part. Such is the case for the azobenzenearsenate (ABA) groups coupled to a polyamino acid carrier. ABA-polytyrosine conjugates show strong delayed hypersensitivity to the hapten but no specificity towards the carrier (Leskowitz, 1963a).

Delayed hypersensitivity response to immunization by hapten-protein conjugates is a complex phenomenon involving three main categories of antigenic determinants (Leskowitz, 1963b):

1. Those produced or revealed in the protein carrier by chemical manipulation,
2. Those consisting of hapten plus the amino acids immediately adjoining its site of attachment,
3. The hapten alone, e.g., the ABA group.

The dual facet of the anamnestic response in delayed hypersensitivity directed against the carrier or the hapten is a manifestation of cellular specificity. A population of B cells with an increased reactivity against the hapten or T cells with an increased sensitivity against the carrier can, at least in part, explain the dual aspect of the response to carrier-hapten conjugates (Mitchison, 1971a,b).

DNP-skin protein conjugates prepared in vivo by painting guinea pigs with 1-fluoro-2,4-dinitrobenzene (DNFB) or 1-chloro-2,4-dinitrobenzene (DNCB) have been shown to be suitable antigens capable of inducing a state of delayed hypersensitivity as assayed by epicutaneous testing of animals injected with the DNP-protein conjugate (McFarlin and Balfour, 1973; Nakagawa and Tanioku, 1972; Nishioka et al., 1971; Parker and Turk, 1970; Parker et al., 1970). DNP-skin protein conjugates can also stimulate (in vitro) human lymphocytes from donors sensitized to DNFB (Milner, 1974) or show migration inhibition factor (MIF) activity in the case of guinea pigs sensitized to DNCB (Camm et al., 1975). Guinea pig skin protein conjugates of the naturally occurring hapten prepared in vitro have also been shown to induce contact sensitivity to the hapten (alantolactone) in guinea pigs. Cross-reactivity to natural and synthetic α-methylene-γ-butyrolactones was observed (Dupuis et al., 1980).

Whole blood cells have been used as hapten carrier. DNCB coupled to erythrocytes or leukocytes yields an antigen capable of inducing lymphocyte transformation and lymphokine production in in vitro cultures of human lymphocytes (Geczy and Baumgarten, 1970; Levis et al., 1975).

The exact nature of the in vivo carrier(s) in allergic contact dermatitis (ACD) remains, however, to be firmly established. The system may be composed of several components: haptenated epidermal, dermal, or serum proteins, and haptenated blood cells. Phagocytic cells may also be implicated, especially in view of their role in antigen "processing."

Synthetic Polymers Used as Carriers

The use of synthetic polymers of amino acids and/or their conjugates has proved to be a valuable tool in the study of the molecular basis of immune phenomena. Such studies have provided a better understanding of delayed hypersensitivity (Borek, 1968), immunologic tolerance (Bauminger et al., 1967; Bauminger and Sela, 1969; Maurer et al., 1965; Sela, 1966), antigenic competition (Ben-Efraim and Liacopoulos, 1967; Schechter, 1968), and genetic control of the immune response (Benacerraf and Dord, 1974; Ben-Efraim et al., 1967; Levine et al., 1963; McDevitt and Sela, 1965; McDevitt and Tyan, 1968; Mozes, 1974; Rathburn and Hildemann, 1970; Rüde and Günther, 1974).

The study of synthetic polymers used as carriers has been mainly limited to the use of polylysine, copolymers of polylysine, and polytyrosine. Such polymers have been used as carriers of various haptens, mainly the DNP group (Yaron et al., 1974) and the ABA group (Collotti and Leskowitz, 1970; Leskowitz, 1963a). From these studies, the following observations have been made:

1. The minimum length of the carrier molecule capable to act as an immunogen or to elicit delayed hypersensitivity is composed of seven to eight amino acid residues (Schlossman et al., 1966) in the case of polylysine.
2. Shorter polypeptides are not immunogenic, but are able to elicit type III (Arthus-type) reactions, i.e., they can react with preformed antibodies (Schlossman and Levine, 1967).
3. Copolymers of lysine and alanine containing five lysine residues (of which four are in a continuous sequence) possess the same immunologic properties as octalysine (Yaron et al., 1974). This observation suggests that immunogenicity is not dependent of an unbroken sequence of lysine residues.
4. The configuration of the amino acids composing the primary structure of the carrier is important. Strain 2 guinea pigs can be sensitized to α,N-DNP-poly-L-lysine (containing 80 residues) but they do not develop delayed or immediate sensitivity when D-lysine replaces L-lysine in the DNP polymer (Schlossman et al., 1965; Ben-Efraim et al., 1967).
5. Changing the conformation of one lysine residue of α,N-DNP-L-polylysine (containing 9 residues) in position 5, produces a peptide that does not

possess immunologic properties. If, however, the D-lysine residue is introduced in position 2 (DNP-L-Lys-D-Lys-L-Lys$_7$), the resulting peptide is
immunologically active (Schlossman and Yaron, 1970). These results have
been interpreted to suggest that the receptor for antigens is highly stereo-
specific.
6. In vitro studies using DNP coupled to octadecalysine (L-Lys$_{18}$) show that
   DNP attached to the ϵ-amino group of the C-terminal lysine residue cannot
   inhibit migration of macrophages from guinea pigs sensitized to DNP covalently bound to the N-terminal lysine residue of the octadecapeptide
   (David and Schlossman, 1968).

Haptens Coupled to a Single Amino Acid Residue: The ABA Group

The p-ABA hapten has been coupled to N-acetyl tyrosine and the compound
obtained has been shown to be a strong immunogen capable of inducing a
relatively pure state of delayed hypersensitivity (Sefik et al., 1972). The delayed reaction is directed against the ABA group with a possible minor contribution by the aromatic phenolic ring of the carrier (Leskowitz et al., 1966,
1970).

It has been found that ABA-acetyltyrosine is less efficient than ABA conjugated to a protein carrier in detecting delayed hypersensitivity in guinea pigs,
presumably because of a faster disappearance of ABA-tyrosine as compared
with ABA-albumin, in intradermal tissues. The conjugates showed, however,
the same activity when assayed in vitro for inhibition of macrophage migration (Nauceil and Raynaud, 1971).

Structure-immunogenicity relationships have been carried out by modification of the stereochemistry or the nature of the amino acid to which the ABA
group is attached and by using various carriers. A study (Hanna and Leskowitz,
1973a,b) of the immunogenicity (ability to sensitize) of various analogs, as
compared with ABA-acetyltyrosine, showed that removal of acetyl group decreased the activity 10 times. The presence of the α-amino group was shown
to be essential, since its removal brought about a 100 X decrease in immunogenicity. The presence of the carboxyl function of the conjugate appeared to
be necessary. Removal of the carboxyl group or its replacement by an amide
function resulted in a decrease in immunogenicity. Simultaneous removal of
the amine and carboxyl functions abolished immunogenicity.

The stereochemistry of the tyrosine moiety did not appear to be of critical
importance since ABA-acetyl-D-tyrosine was as effective as the L-isomer in

eliciting sensitization (Hanna et al., 1973). This latter result would suggest that metabolic "processing" of this conjugate is not essential.

Studies of these various analogs in vitro using the lymphocyte (guinea pig) transformation test showed results similar to the in vivo reaction (Hanna et al., 1973). The highest stimulation was obtained with ABA-acetyl-L-tyrosine. The tyrosinamide analog was equally as effective. ABA-acetyl-L-tyramine and ABA-tyrosine were significantly less effective. Total loss of stimulation was observed when the amino and carboxyl groups were removed. Additional studies (Nauciel, 1972) showed that the ABA group is immunodominant and that lymphoid cells can distinguish between various ABA-amino acid conjugates, although part of the recognition system implies part of the amino acid. Lymphocytes from guinea pigs sensitized to ABA-acetyl-L-tyrosine could be stimulated by ABA-acetyl-L-tyrosine but not by ABA-acetyl-L-tryptophan. The presence of macrophages in these cultures was required. Treatment of the cultures with carrageenan, a substance that kills macrophages, decreased stimulation. This last observation suggests a possible "processing" role by phagocytic cells, in contrast with the results cited above, in the case of the ability of the conjugate to induce sensitization.

ABA-tyrosine appears to possess the properties of a "complete" antigen and thus can serve as carrier for macromolecular polypeptides such as ribonuclease A, guinea pig albumin, and bovine albumin. The delayed hypersensitive reaction observed in these cases appeared to be directed towards the hapten (ABA) rather than the macromolecular carrier (Alkan et al., 1972).

The chemical structures of various ABA-tyrosine derivatives discussed above are shown in Figure 1.

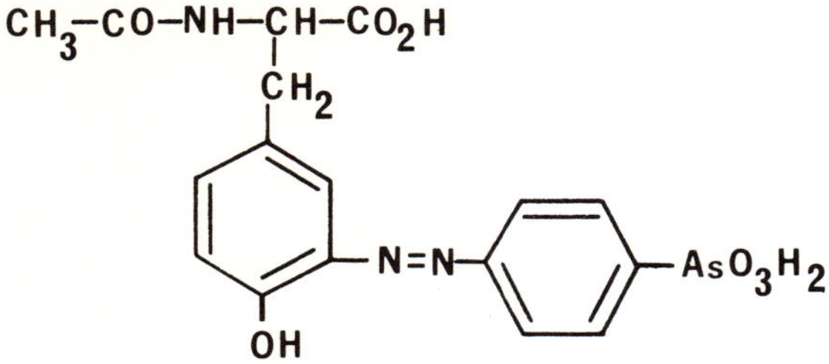

N-acetyl-tyrosine-p-azobenzenearsonic acid

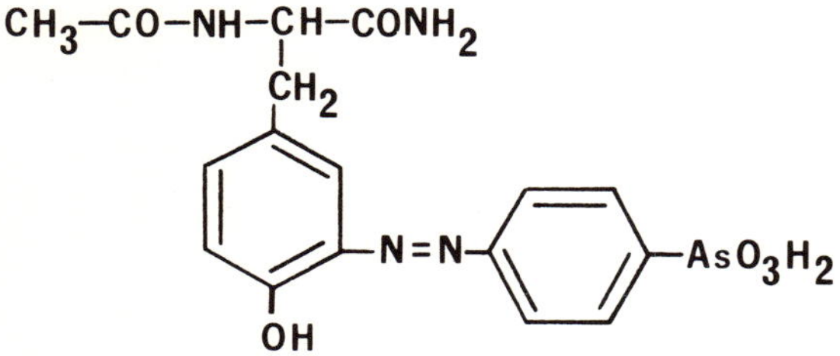

N-acetyl-tyrosinamide-p-azobenzenearsonic acid

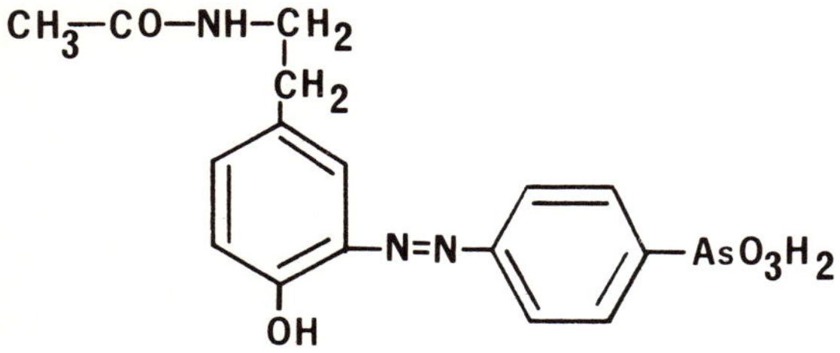

N-acetyl-p-tyramine-p-azobenzenearsonic acid

Figure 1 Chemical structures of various ABA-tyrosine derivatives and analogs.

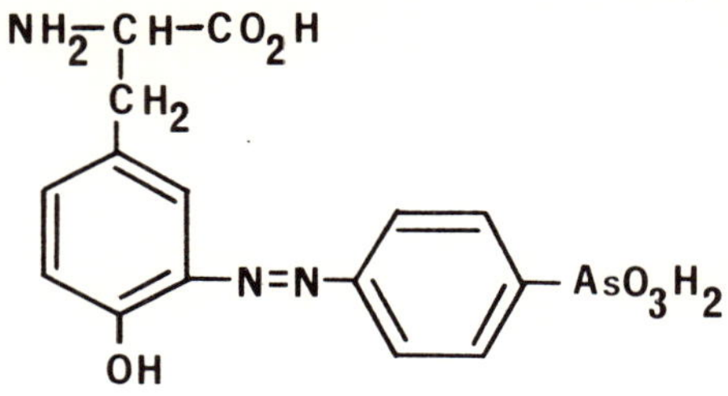

tyrosine-p-azobenzenearsonic acid

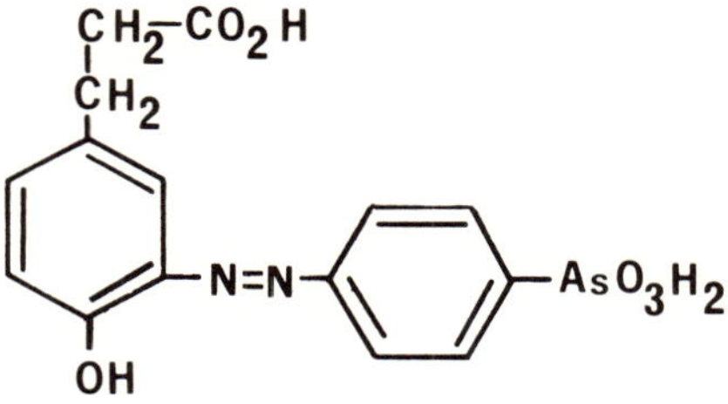

phloretic acid-p-azobenzenearsonic acid

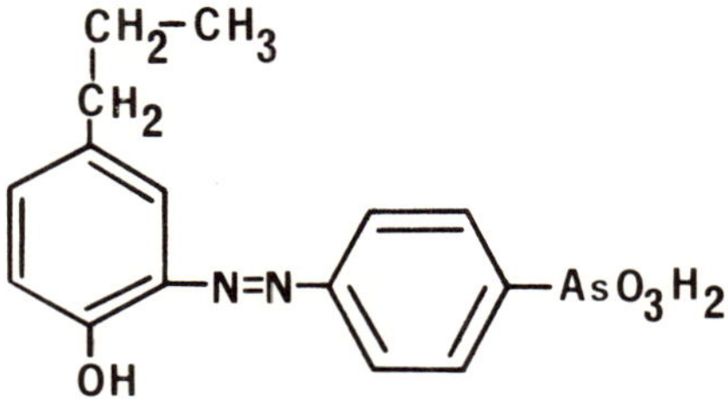

3-propylphenol-p-azobenzenearsonic acid

Figure 1 (continued)

5

Nature of Hapten-Protein Interactions

Allergic contact dermatitis (ACD) to simple chemicals results from (selective) cellular recognition of a hapten-carrier conjugate. It is, therefore a propos to review the types of chemical bonds that can occur between the two reactants, hapten and carrier. There are two broad classes of chemical bonds: covalent bonds and ionic bonds.

In *covalent bonds,* an electron pair represented by — is shared by the hapten (H) and the carrier (C):

$$H + C \longrightarrow H-C$$

According to the nature of the carrier, several covalent bonds can be formed. Covalent bonds are strong and require large amounts of energy to be broken.

Ionic (electrostatic) bonds are formed by coulombic attraction between reactants bearing electrostatic charges of opposite sign. This can be illustrated by:

$$H^+ + C^- \longrightarrow H-C \quad ; \quad H^- + C^+ \longrightarrow H-C$$

C and/or H may or may not bear a formal charge but instead, due to the existence of dipoles, a partial positive or negative charge. This can be illustrated by an electrostatic interaction (hydrogen bond) between an alcohol (R–OH) and a ketone (R–C–R),
$$\underset{O}{\overset{\|}{}}$$

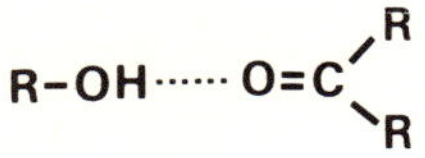

$$R-OH \cdots\cdots O=C \begin{smallmatrix} R \\ \diagup \\ \diagdown \\ R \end{smallmatrix} \qquad \text{(hydrogen bond)}$$

or the interaction of a copper salt (Cu^{++}) with a diamine.

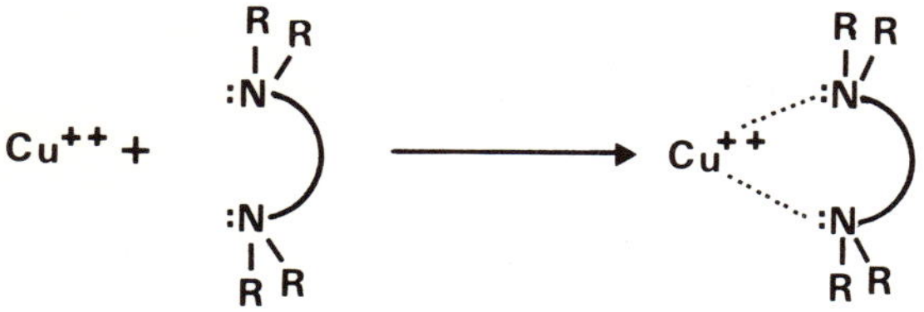

The nature of the in vivo carrier remains to be firmly established. It is likely, however, that proteins play a dominant role in formation of the antigen involved in ACD. The following discussion is an attempt to clarify the nature of covalent and electrostatic bonds between haptens and proteins.

Classification of Organic Reactions

Covalent Bonds

Most chemical reactions can be described as being the attack of an electron-deficient species on an electron-rich entity. Electron pairs (or doublets) are involved. An electron-deficient species is an electrophile ("electron seeking" entity). There are several examples, which include:

1. Positively charged species (*cations*) such as protons (H^+), metal salts, (Cu^{++}, Ni^{++}, etc.), quaternary ammonium salts (R_4N^+), etc.
2. Molecules possessing unsaturated bonds (double or triple bonds) conjugated with an electron-withdrawing group

$$H_2C = CH - CO_2 - C_2H_5$$

ethyl acrylate

3. Aromatic compounds possessing electron-withdrawing groups

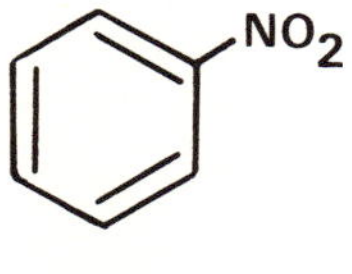

nitrobenzene

4. Centers bearing a strongly electronegative atom

(δ indicates a partial positive or negative charge)

$$\overset{\delta^+}{-CH_2}\overset{\delta^-}{-Br} \quad ; \quad \overset{\delta^+}{-C}\overset{\delta^-}{=O}$$

5. Transient species (not to be discussed here) such as carbenes, $R_2C:$ (divalent carbon), nitrenes, $RN:$ (monovalent nitrogen), etc.

An electron-rich species is a *nucleophile.* there are numerous examples, including:

1. Negatively charged species (anions)

$$H_5C_2CO_2CH_2^- \quad ; \quad R-S^- \quad ; \quad R-O^- \quad ; \quad R_2N^- \quad ; \quad etc.$$

2. An atom possessing one or more unshared electron pairs (doublets)

$$R_3N: \quad ; \quad R-\ddot{O}-R \quad ; \quad R-\ddot{S}-R \quad ; \quad etc.$$

There are also reactions that involve only *one* electron. These reactions are *radical* reactions. The presence of light or of a radical initiator (e.g., a peroxide) is required. The chemical species involved are one-electron entities.

$$R^\bullet \; ; \; R-O^\bullet \; ; \; R-S^\bullet \; ; \; etc.$$

Two-electron Reactions

These chemical reactions can be divided into *nucleophilic* and *electrophilic* substitutions and *nucleophilic* addition.

Nucleophilic substitution (S_N) can occur at:

1. A saturated atomic center. In this case, no double bonds are involved and there is a direct substitution of one atom (or a group of atoms) by the incoming nucleophile.

2. An unsaturated atomic center. In this instance, multiple bonds are in-

involved. Addition-elimination occurs, resulting in a net substitution.

Electrophilic substitution (S_E) is the result of interaction of an electron-deficient species with an electron-rich species,

(electrophile)

where E^+ is an electrophile such as H^+, NO_2^+, Br^+, etc.

Nucleophilic addition on unsaturated systems. In this case, the electron-rich species is the nucleophile and the unsaturated system is the electrophile. The reaction results in formation of a saturated compound.

$$R-\ddot{N}H_2 + CH_2=CH-COOR' \longrightarrow R-NH-CH_2-CH_2-COOR'$$
(nucleophile)   (electrophile)

One-electron Reactions

These reactions involve *radicals*.

Very often, in ACD, R is a halogen.

Electrostatic Bonds

These chemical bonds play an essential role in biological systems. Hydrogen bonds, salt-bridge formation, hydrophobic and weak (van der Waals' type) interactions are, in large part, responsible for maintaining conformation, structure, and activity of enzymes, proteins, nucleic acids, cellular membranes, etc.

in living organisms (Pauling, 1960; Tanford, 1973; Watson, 1977). These interactions are, in general, weak ones that can be broken at a small expense of energy. The presence of a large number of these interactions in a given (macro) molecule can result in a very stable structure, e.g., base pairing in deoxyribonucleic acids (DNAs). The relevance of these interactions to ACD will be discussed in the next section.

Chemical Reactions between Haptens and Proteins

Proteins possess several functional groups (side chains) that can act as *nucleophiles*. The most important ones include the ϵ-amino group of lysine residues, the sulfhydryl group of cysteine residues, and the imidazole group of histidine residues.

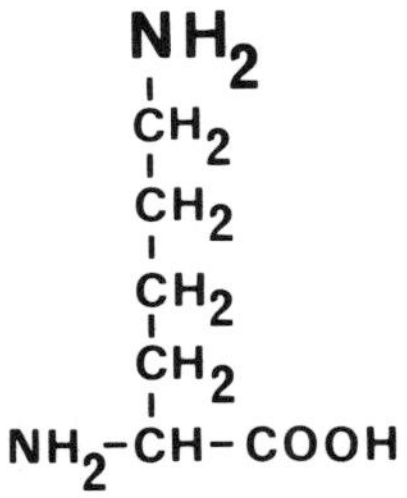

$$
\begin{array}{ccc}
\text{lysine} & \text{cysteine} & \text{histidine}
\end{array}
$$

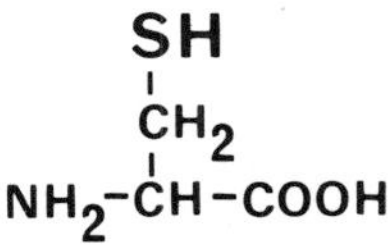

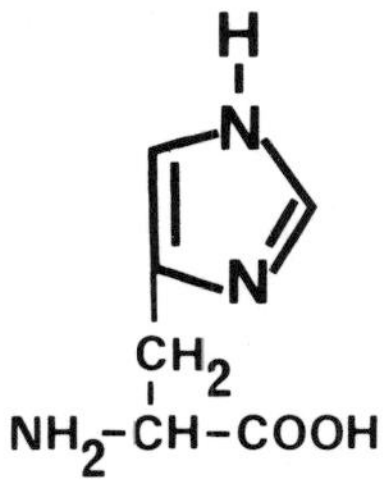

Other groups, such as the hydroxyl group of serine and the thioether function of methionine residues, are poorer nucleophiles and they need a special environment and spatial arrangements of atoms (conformation) to be involved in nucleophilic reactions. These requirements are fulfilled in enzymes such as serine proteases (James, 1980) or in the formation of S-adenosyl methionine, a donor of one carbon unit in metabolic reactions.

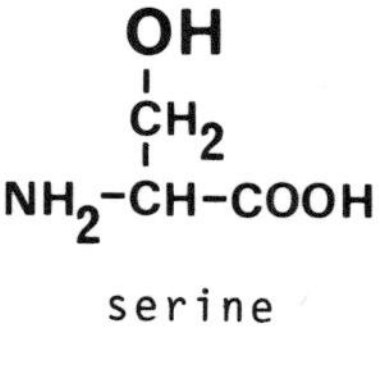

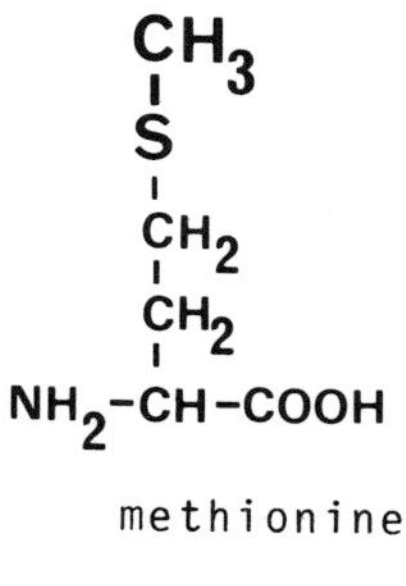

Aromatic groups in proteins can be involved in radical reactions.

Most of the known *haptens* (H) involved in ACD, possess electron-deficient centers. They are, therefore, electrophiles and can be attacked by the nucleophilic groups of protein side chains. Certain haptens also possess labile (usually carbon-halogen) bonds, which can be broken to form radicals able to react with unsaturated (aromatic) sites in proteins.

Two-electron Reactions

Nucleophilic substitution at a *saturated* center can be exemplified by the reaction of ω-chloroacetophenone with the ε-amino group of a lysine residue.

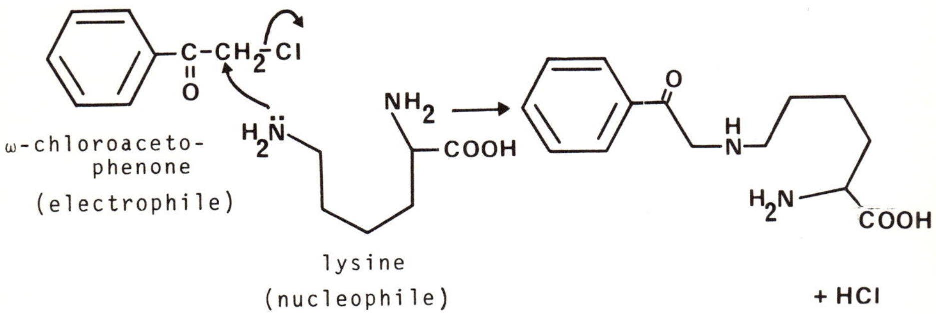

Nucleophilic substitution at an *unsaturated* center can be exemplified by reaction of 1-fluoro-2,4-dinitrobenzene (DNFB) with the ε-amino group of lysine.

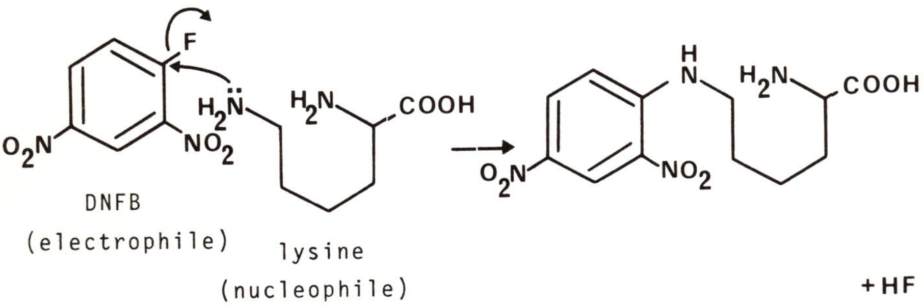

Nucleophilic addition to an *unsaturated* center can be illustrated by the reaction of alantolactone, a sesquiterpene α-methylene-γ-butyrolactone, with cysteine (Dupuis et al., 1974). The nucleophile is the thiol group (SH) of cysteine.

alantolactone
(electrophile)

cysteine
(nucleophile)

The reactions mentioned above can proceed under physiological conditions, as has been shown in the case of sesquiterpene lactones (Dupuis et al., 1974; Kupchan et al., 1970); here adducts are obtained in phosphate buffer at pH 5.4 or 7.4. In addition, these terpenes can react with ribonuclease A or with skin proteins (Dupuis et al., 1980). Halogenated dinitrobenzene derivatives such as DNFB and 1-chloro-2,4-dinitrobenzene (DNCB) can also react with proteins under physiological conditions (Eisen, 1964).

Electrophilic substitution can be exemplified by the reaction of azobenzene-arsonate (ABA) with tyrosine.

ABA   tyrosine

This reaction has been shown to proceed under physiological conditions (Collotti and Leskowitz, 1970). The diazo derivative is prepared by reacting the *para*-amino compound with nitrous acid prior to coupling.

One-electron Reactions

One-electron reactions can be illustrated by reaction of 3,3′,4,5′-tetrachloro-salicylanilide (TCSA; Irgasan BS200) with a tyrosine residue.
  Light irradiation of TCSA produces two radicals.

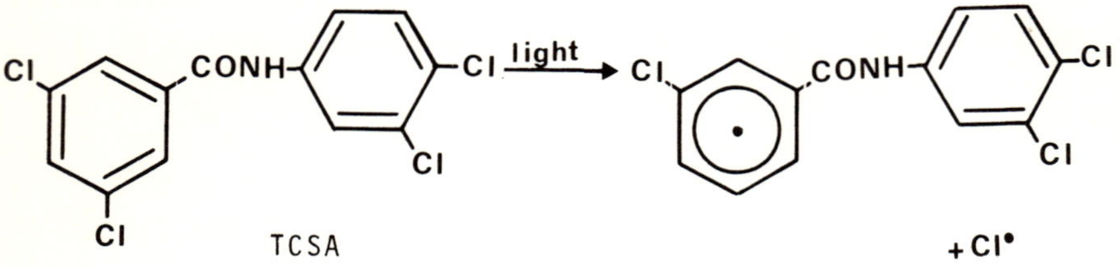

Reaction of the free radical TCSA with a tyrosine residue gives

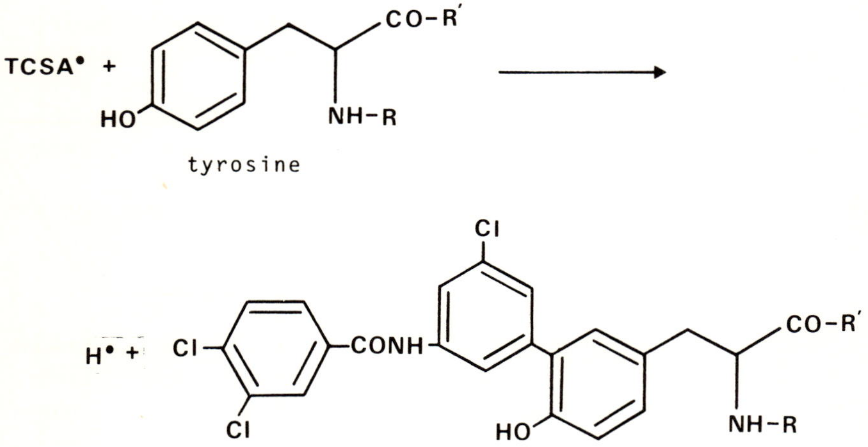

The overall reaction can thus be written as:

TCSA + tyrosine residue → TCSA – tyrosine residue + HCl

Electrostatic Interactions

Salt-bridge Formation

Hapten-carrier adduct can also result from electrostatic interactions between species of opposite charges. Such interactions can be exemplified by salt-bridge formation between quaternary ammonium salt and the carboxylic side chains of aspartic and glutamic acid residues in proteins.

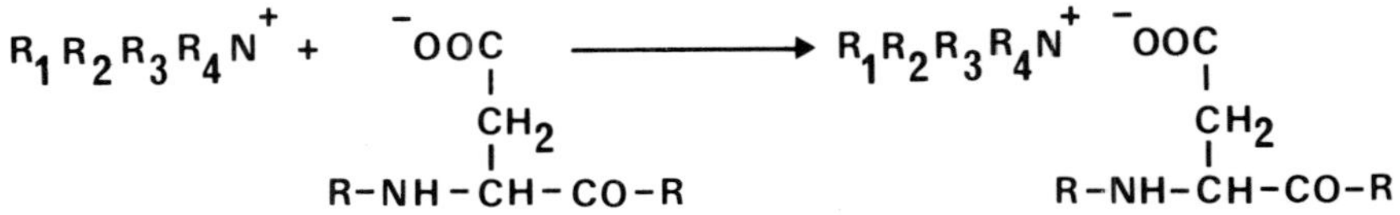

$$R_1R_2R_3R_4\overset{+}{N} + \;\;\overset{-}{OOC} \longrightarrow R_1R_2R_3R_4\overset{+}{N}\;\;\overset{-}{OOC}$$

$$\begin{array}{cc} & | \\ & CH_2 \\ & | \\ R-NH-CH-CO-R \end{array} \qquad \begin{array}{cc} & | \\ & CH_2 \\ & | \\ R-NH-CH-CO-R \end{array}$$

Formation of Complexes

Coordination compounds (complexes) can be formed by filling unoccupied orbitals of an acceptor with electron pairs from a donor.

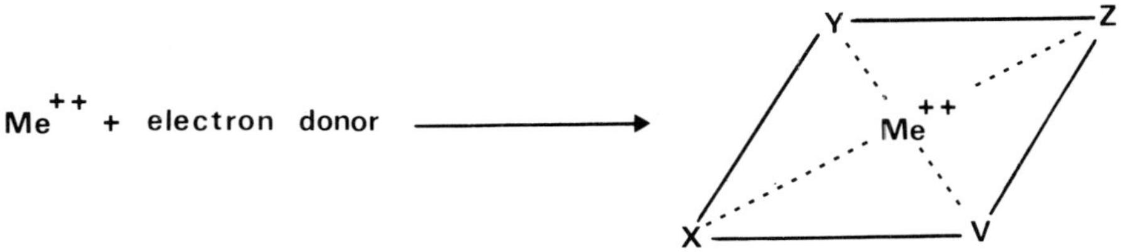

$$Me^{++} + electron\;\; donor \longrightarrow$$

In the above equation, a metal with a positive charge forms four coordinate bonds with four electron donors (N, X, Y, Z). Examples of coordinate compounds common in nature include, for example, magnesium (Mg^{++}) in chlorophyll, cobalt (Co^{6+}) in vitamin B_{12}, etc.

6

Chemically Reactive Functions in Haptens and in Proteins

Amino Acids

Sensitization and immunological reactions to haptens in allergic contact dermatitis (ACD) to simple chemicals is the result of an immune response directed towards the hapten combined with the carrier molecule*. The nature of the in vivo carrier is still not precisely known, although it is very likely that the immunogen is the result of reaction of the hapten with a specific protein or with soluble or cellular proteins.

The structure of the in vivo antigen will depend on the chemical properties of the hapten and also on the amino acid composition and the primary, secondary, tertiary, and, perhaps, quaternary structure of the carrier.

To illustrate this point, let us consider two haptens, 1-fluoro-2,4-dinitrobenzene (DNFB) and 3,3',4,5'-tetrachlorosalicylanilide (TCSA), with unrelated chemically reactive groups. DNFB can undergo a nucleophilic displacement at carbon one in the presence of a nucleophile (see Chap. 5) to yield the corresponding dinitrophenyl (DNP) derivative. In proteins, substitution will occur mainly on the side chain of tyrosine, lysine, and cysteine residues. The degree

---

*For the purpose of discussion of amino acid reactivity, we have assumed that the in vivo carrier is proteinic in nature and that polysaccharides, nucleic acids, or complex lipids play a minor role in ACD to simple chemicals, if any. In the remaining discussion, the term "carrier" will be used in a broad sense without necessarily meaning a unique molecular species.

of hapten substitution will thus depend on the number and accessibility of these amino acid residues. In addition, the positions of the reactive amino acids will also determine the positions of the hapten and the distance between the substituted positions. The nature of the amino acid residues adjacent to the substituted tyrosine, lysine, or cysteine may also contribute to the immune response.

Similar considerations can be put forward in the case of TCSA. In this case, however, the resulting antigen will be of a different nature. TCSA forms radicals (see Chap. 5) when exposed to sunlight or other light sources of high energy. Such a radical will seek an electron-deficient system. In this instance, most probable reactions will occur with tyrosine, phenylalanine, tryptophan, and histidine side chains.

Obviously DNFB and TCSA will form chemically and immunologically different antigens. It cannot be excluded, however, that the same protein can serve as carrier in either example. Only the nature of the resulting antigen will be different.

Proteins are made of 20 different α-amino acids. Each amino acid possesses at least two reactive functional groups, an amino and a carboxyl group. Since these two functions are, in proteins, involved in peptide (amide) bonds, only amino acids possessing a chemically reactive side chain will be involved in reactions with haptens. These various amino acids are illustrated in Table 1.

Nucleophilic Amino Acids

Amino acids possessing a sulfhydryl (SH), amino (NH_2), or imidazole group can act as nucleophiles (see Chap. 5). In this respect, cysteine (–SH), lysine (–NH_2), and histidine (imidazole) are good candidates for nucleophilic reactivity.

Since thiols (R–SH) are among the best known nucleophiles, cysteine will be a good candidate for reaction with haptens. Primary amines are strong nucleophiles; therefore, the ϵ-amino group of lysine will also be involved in nucleophilic reactions. Nucleophilic reactions involving imidazoles are also possible, although the ring nitrogens are weaker nucleophiles than amines. The two nitrogens are not equivalent: the "tele" nitrogen is approximately three times more reactive than the "pro" nitrogen (Wieghardt and Goren, 1975).

Table 1 List of the Commonly Occurring Amino Acids Which May Be Implicated in Chemical Reactions with Haptens in ACD

Amino acids	Abbreviations[a]	Structure of the side chain (R)[b]
Arginine	Arg (R)	$NH_2-C-NH-(CH_2)_3-$ $\quad\quad\quad\,\,$NH
Aspartic acid	Asp (D)	HO_2C-CH_2-
Cysteine	Cys (C)	$HS-CH_2-$
Glutamic acid	Glu (E)	$HO_2C-CH_2-CH_2-$
Histidine	His (H)	(imidazole)$-CH_2^-$
Lysine	Lys (K)	$NH_2-(CH_2)_4-$
Methionine	Met (M)	$CH_3-S-CH_2-CH_2-$
Phenylalanine	Phe (F)	(phenyl)$-CH_2^-$
Serine	Ser (S)	$HO-CH_2-$
Threonine	Thr (T)	$CH_3-CH(OH)-$
Tryptophan	Trp (W)	(indolyl)$-CH_2^-$
Tyrosine	Tyr (Y)	$HO-$(phenyl)$-CH_2^-$

[a]Nomenclature of a-amino acids. Recommendations, 1974. I.U.P.A.C. Commission on the nomenclature of organic chemistry and I.U.P.A.C.-I.U.B. Commission on biochemical nomenclature. *Biochemistry* (1975) *14*, 449-462.

[b]The general formula used is: $NH_2-\overset{\overset{\textstyle R}{|}}{C}H-COOH$.

Primary alcohols (R—OH) are, in general, poor nucleophiles. The hydroxyl group can, however, act as a nucleophile when located in a special environment, as it is in the case of serine residues in certain proteases (James, 1980; Williams, 1969). Nucleophilicity of primary alcohols will be sufficient when they react with a molecule possessing a good leaving group (e.g., opening of an anhydride).

The indolyl side chain of tryptophan can serve as nucleophile and reaction will involve the ring nitrogen, the α- or the β-positions (Woodward et al., 1963). Under physiological conditions, however, these reactions are probably not important.

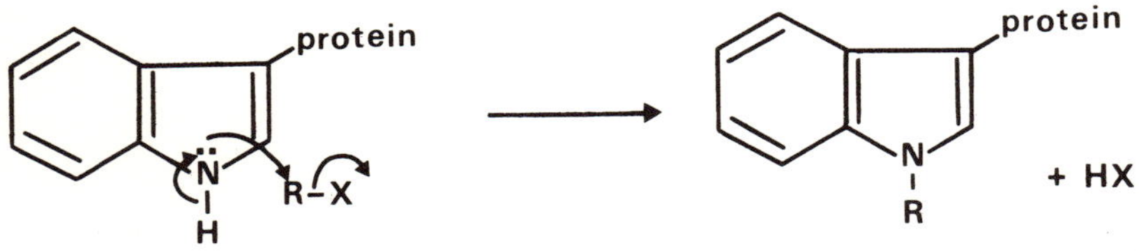

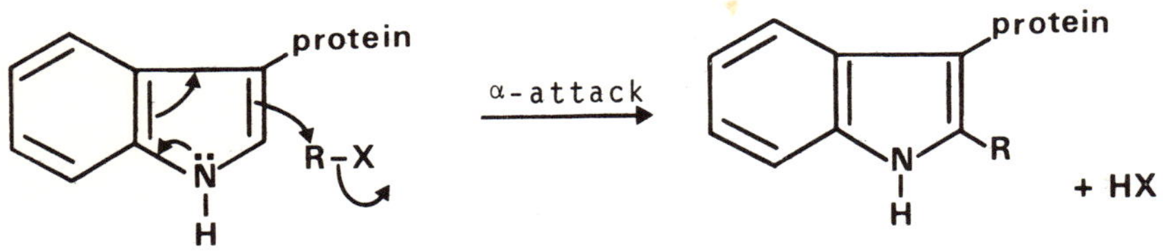

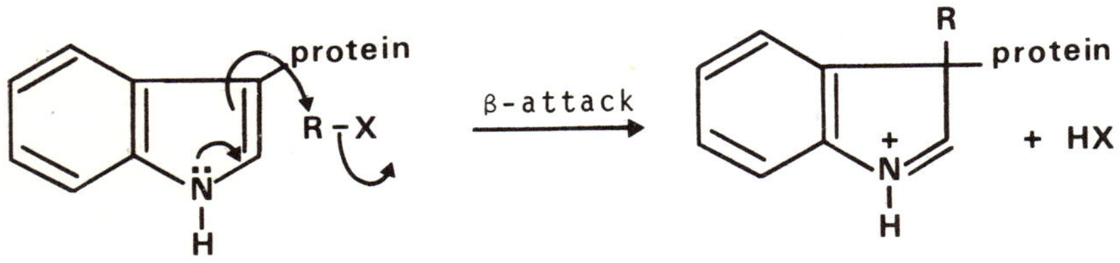

The sulfur atom of methionine can be alkylated by reagents such as cyanogen bromide (Gross and Witkop, 1962) and halogenated acetic acid and its acetate ester or amide (Glick et al., 1967; Neumann et al., 1962). These reactions require, however, particular conditions which, for the purpose of ACD to simple chemicals, make methionine residues poor candidates for nucleophilic attack of the hapten.

The guanido group of arginine is probably a poor nucleophile in vivo because the group still remains strongly protonated at pH 7 to 8 (Greenstein and Winitz, 1961). At pH 7.3, 0.0006% of the guanido group is in its unprotonated (nucleophilic) form.

$$
\begin{array}{c}
NH_2 \\
| \\
C=NH \\
| \\
NH \\
| \\
CH_2 \\
| \\
CH_2 \\
| \\
CH_2 \\
| \\
NH_2-CH-COOH
\end{array}
$$

arginine

Aromatic Amino Acids

The side chain of tyrosine, tryptophan, and phenylalanine can serve as electron acceptors; they will be primarily involved in one-electron reactions (see Chap. 5). Their role will be especially important in cases of photoallergy to chemicals (Herman and Sams, 1972; Jung et al., 1968).

Reaction of a free radical with tyrosine will first occur in the position α to the phenolic group because of the electron-directing effect of the hydroxyl (phenolic) group. Phenylalanine can also react with free radicals. The favored positions are *ortho* and *para* (Wheland and Pauling, 1935), because of lower electronic densities on these carbons. Tryptophan can participate in reactions with free radicals. In this case, the α position is favored (Ohno and Witkop, 1970). Histidine can also trap free radicals because of electron deficiency of its imidazole ring.

Table 2 proposes a classification of the natural amino acids according to their chemical reactivity.

Table 2 Classification of Amino Acids: Nucleophiles and One-electron Acceptors

Nucleophiles	One-electron acceptors
Cysteine	Tyrosine
Lysine	Phenylalanine
Histidine	Tryptophan
Possibly:	Histidine
Serine	
Threonine	
Tryptophan	
Arginine	

Haptens: A Classification of Haptens Based on Their Reactivity

Sources and structures of haptens are extremely variable. These compounds occur in plants, microorganisms, algae, etc. However, the majority of haptens are man-made and are found in industrial products such as rubber, plastics, dyes, detergents, creams, paints, cosmetics, etc. It is also unfortunate that certain substances used as medications may, in some instances, act as strong allergens.

All allergens are not products of synthesis or biosynthesis, and it is well established that simple compounds such as metal salts can cause severe contact allergies. The occurrence and clinical significance of simple chemicals in ACD has been discussed by Foussereau and Benezra (1970, 1982) and Fisher (1973). In addition, a new journal, *Contact Dermatitis,* is specially devoted to ACD.

We shall classify haptens according to their chemical reactivity in relationship to putative carrier proteins.

Group I. Haptens susceptible to nucleophilic substitution at a saturated center (see Chap. 5).
Group II. Haptens susceptible to nucleophilic substitution (S_N) at an unsaturated center (see Chap. 5).
Group III. Haptens susceptible to electrophilic reactions (see Chap. 5).
Group IV. Haptens susceptible to nucleophilic addition (see Chap. 5).
Group V. Haptens susceptible to radical reactions (loss of halogens; see Chap. 5).
Group VI. Haptens susceptible to various nucleophilic reactions—nucleophilic substitution or nucleophilic addition (see Chap. 5).
Group VII. Metallic salts possessing chelating properties.

Table 3 Haptens Susceptible to Nucleophilic Substitution at a Saturated Center (arrow indicates site of attack)

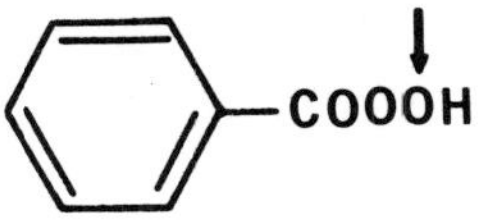

benzoyl peroxide

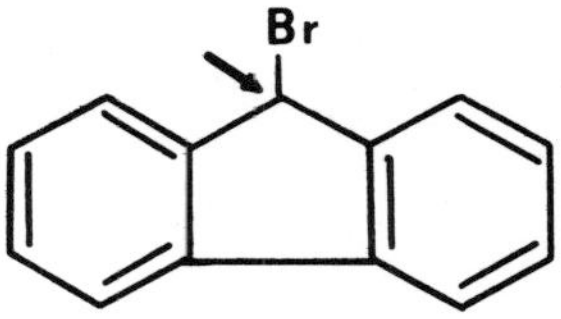

9-bromofluorene

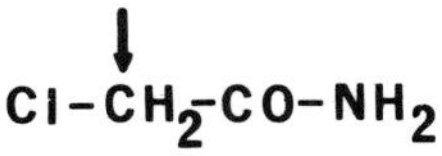

chloroacetamide

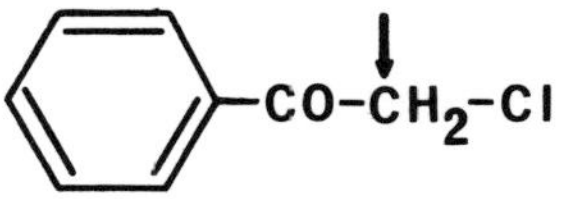

ω-chloroacetophenone

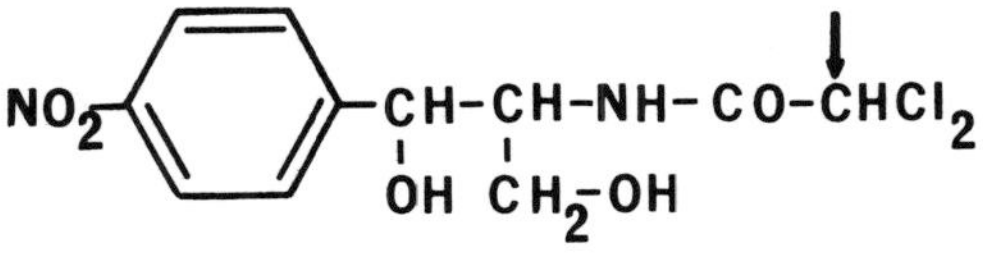

chloramphenicol

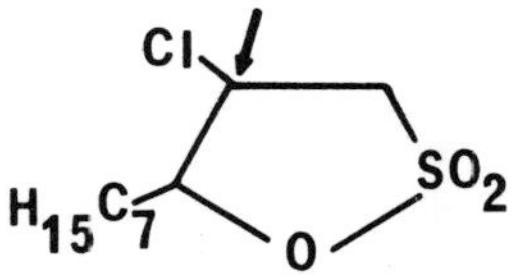

2-chloro-1,3-decanesultone

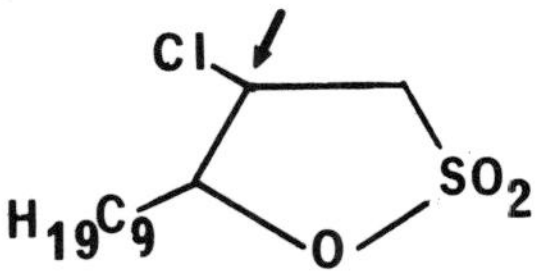

2-chloro-1,3-dodecanesultone

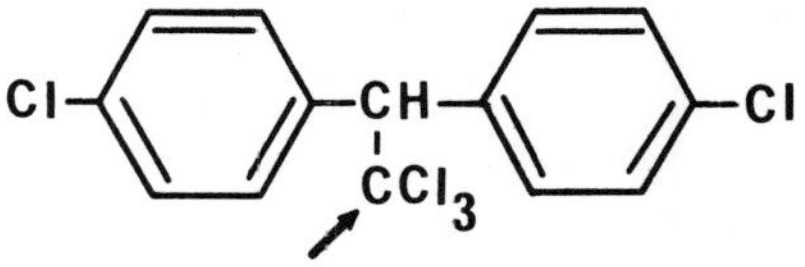

DDT

(continued)

Table 3 (continued)

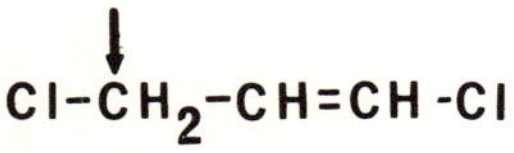

dichlorophene

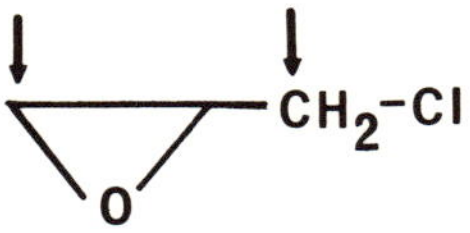

glycerol epichlorhydrin

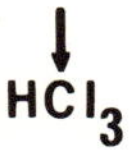

iodoform

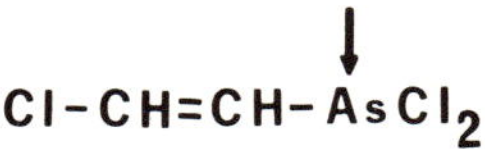

lewisite

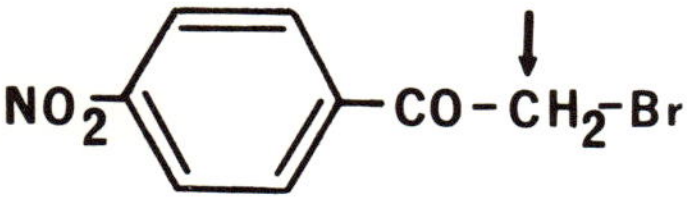

p-nitro-ω-bromoacetophenone

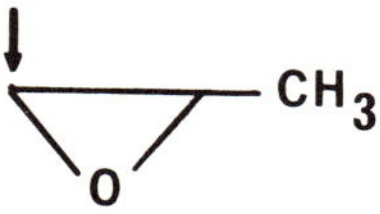

propylene oxide

Table 4 Haptens Susceptible to Nucleophilic Substitution at an Unsaturated
Center (arrow indicates site of attack)

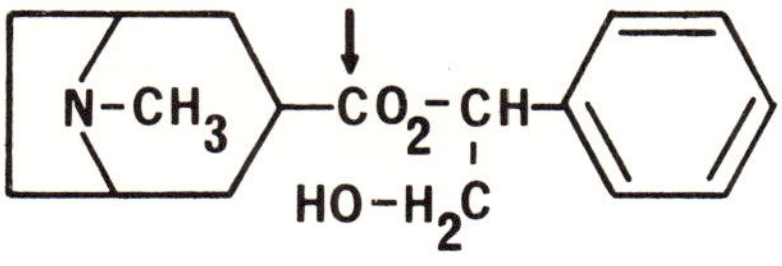

atropine

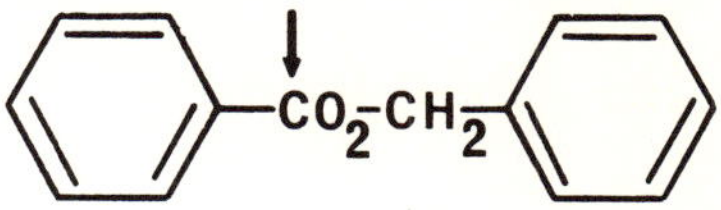

benzyl benzoate

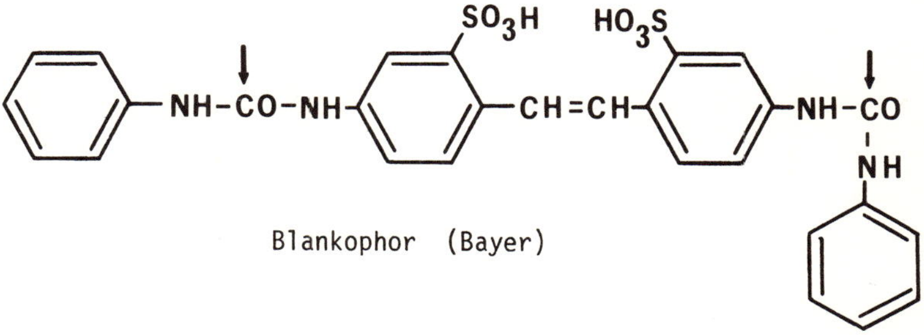

Blankophor   (Bayer)

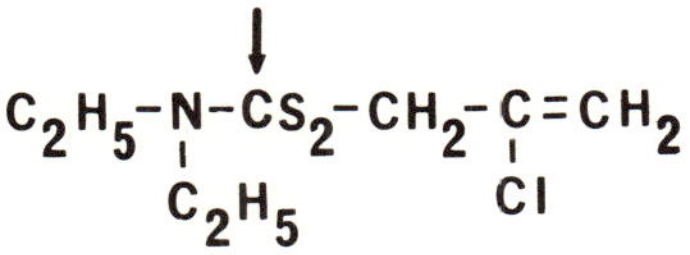

CD-2   (Kodak)

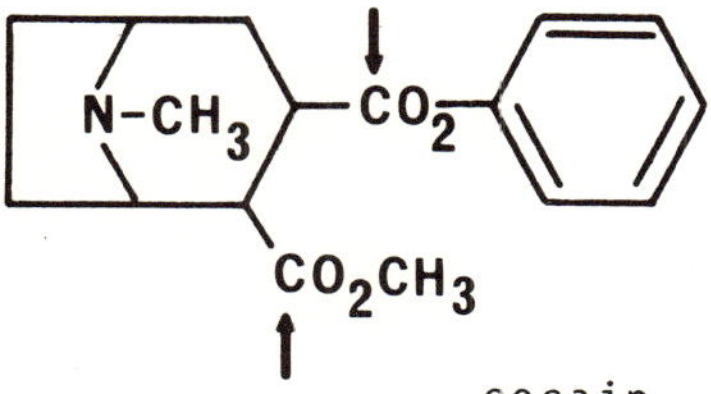

cocain

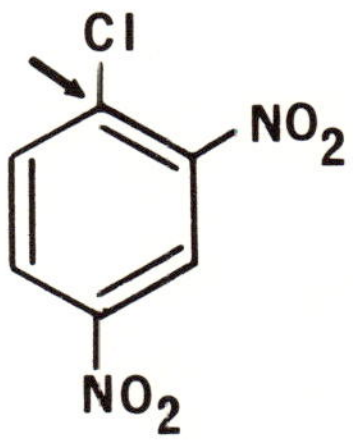

1-chloro-2,4-dinitrobenzene
(DNCB)

(continued)

Table 4 (continued)

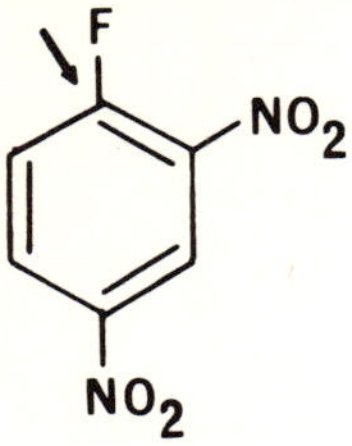

1-fluoro-2,4-dinitrobenzene
(DNFB)

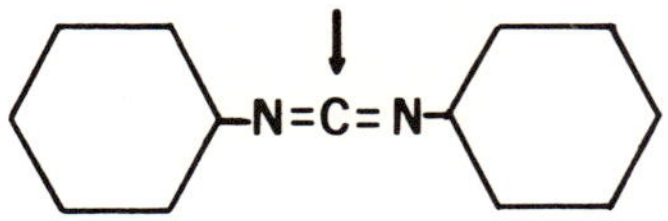

N,N'-dicyclohexylcarbodiimide
(DCC)

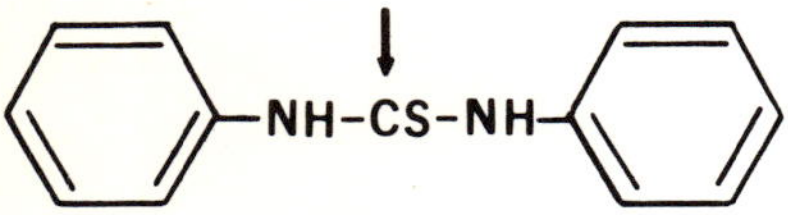

diphenylthiourea

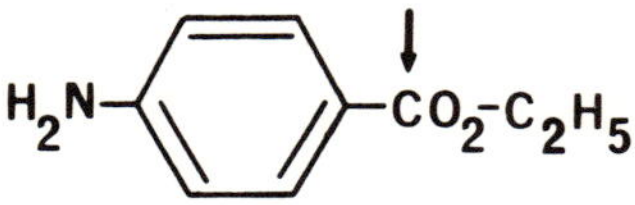

ethyl p-aminobenzoate

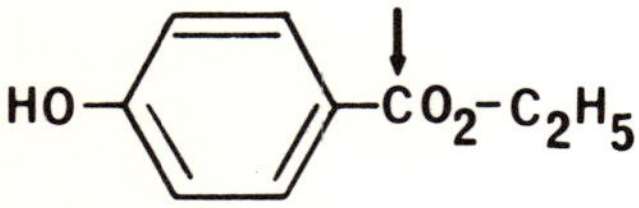

ethyl p-hydroxybenzoate

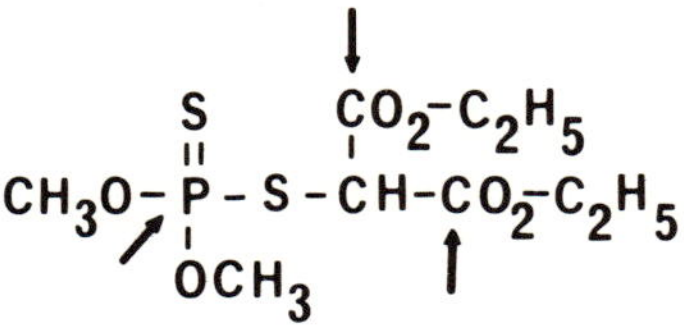

Malathion

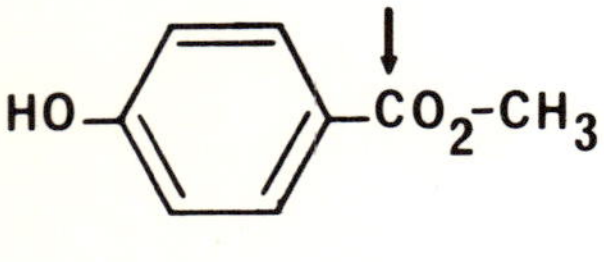

methyl p-hydroxybenzoate

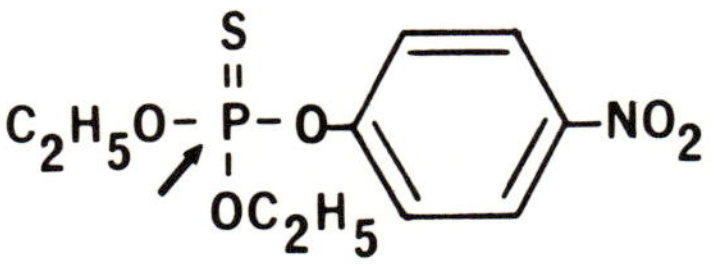

Parathion

(continued)

Table 4 (continued)

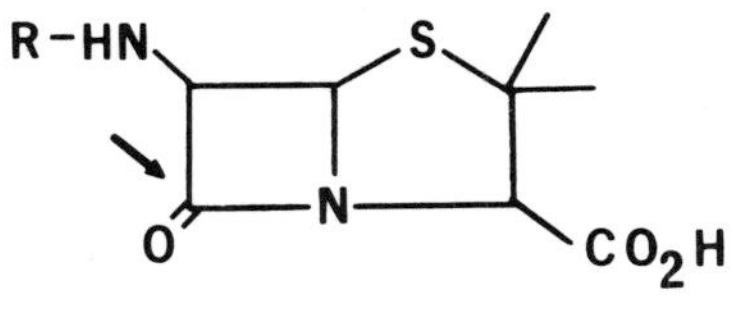

penicillin

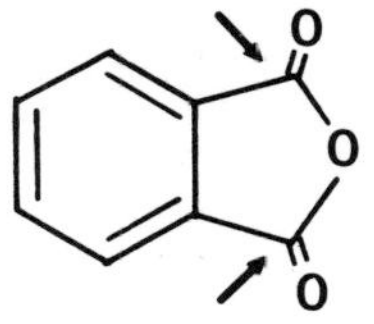

phtalic anhydride

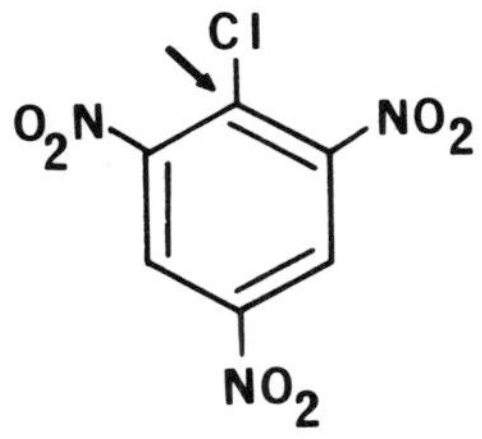

1-chloro-2,4,6-trinitrobenzene
(picryl chloride)

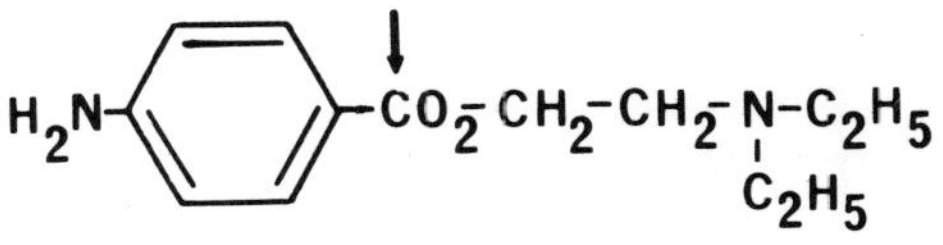

procaine

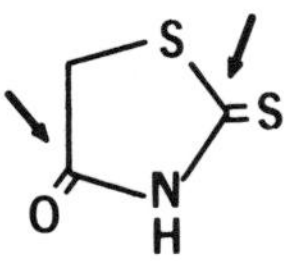

Rhodamin B

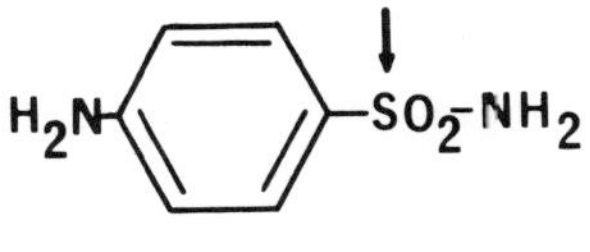

sulfanilamide

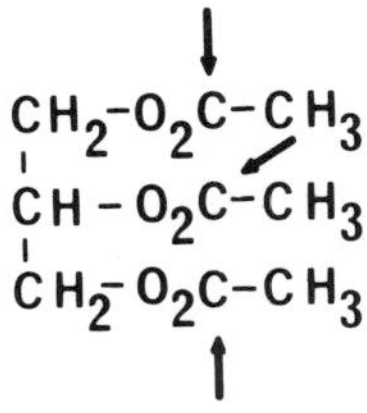

triacetin

Table 5 Haptens Susceptible to Participation in Electrophilic Reactions
(arrow indicates site of attack)

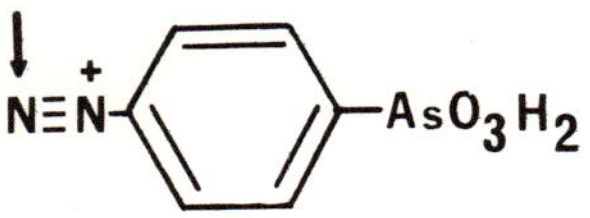

p-aminobenzenearsonate diazonium salt 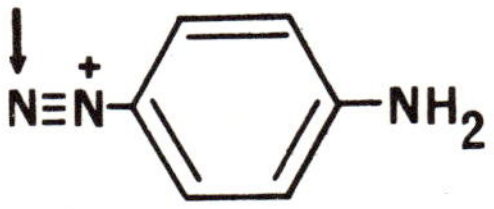   p-aminobenzene diazonium salt

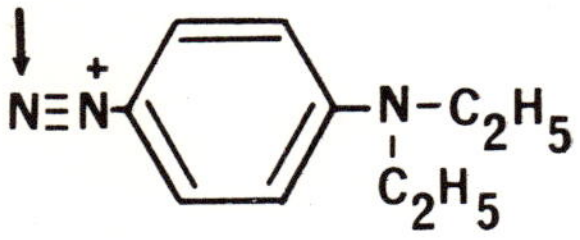

p-diethylaminobenzene diazonium salt

Table 6 Haptens Susceptible to Nucleophilic Addition (arrow indicates site of attack)

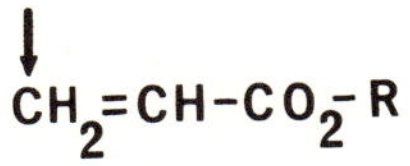

$CH_2=CH-CO_2^- R$

acrylates

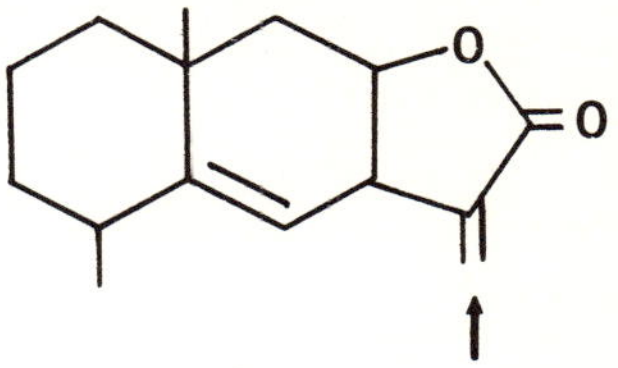

alantolactone

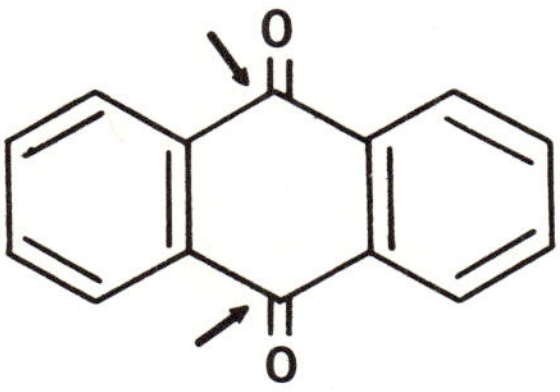

anthraquinone

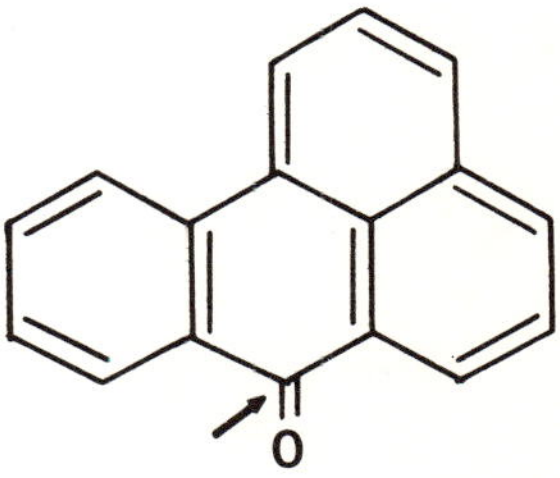

benzanthrone

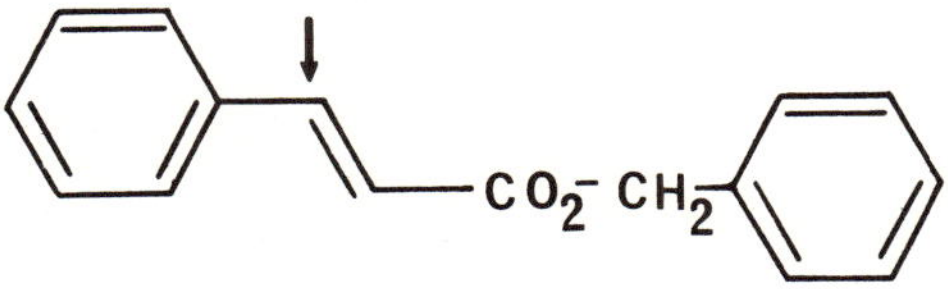

benzyl cinnamate

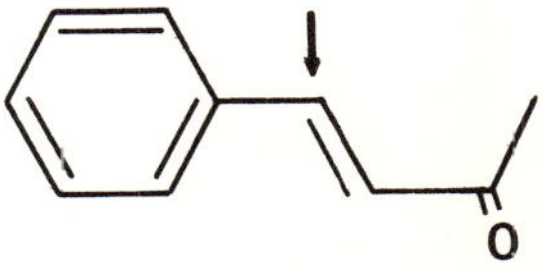

benzylidene acetone

(continued)

Table 6 (continued)

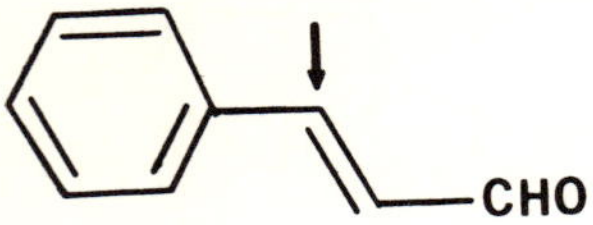

cinnamaldehyde

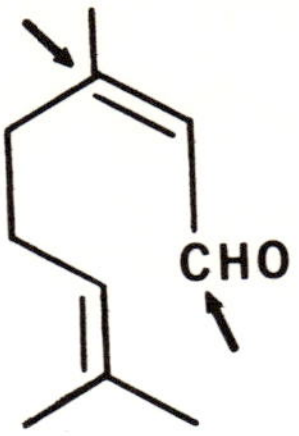

citral

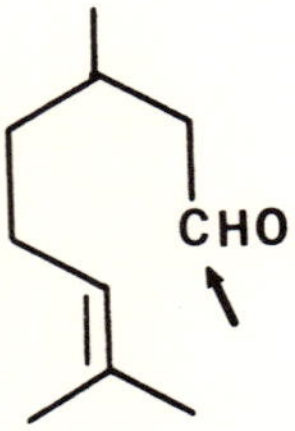

citronellal

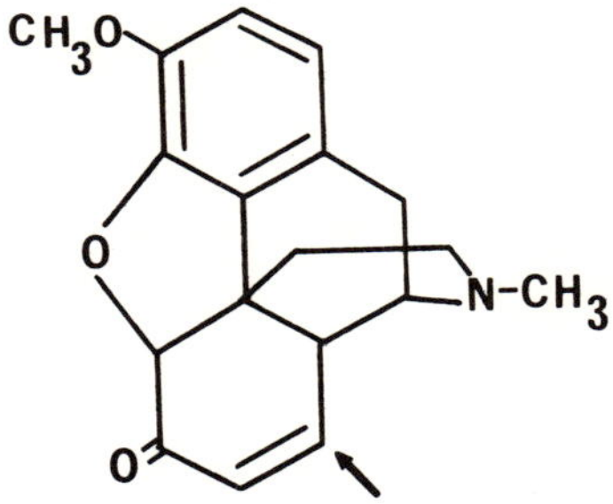

codeinone

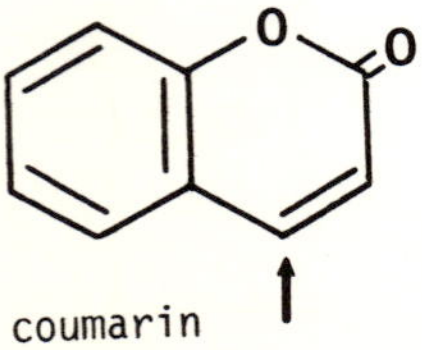

coumarin

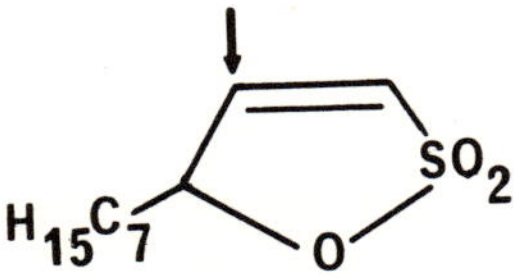

1-decene-1,3-sultone

(continued)

Table 6 (continued)

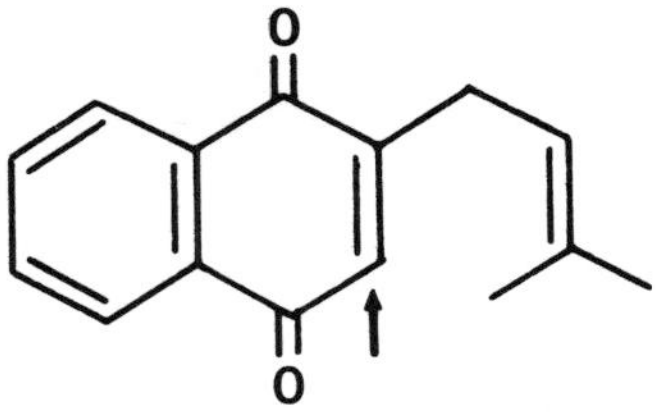

deoxylapachol

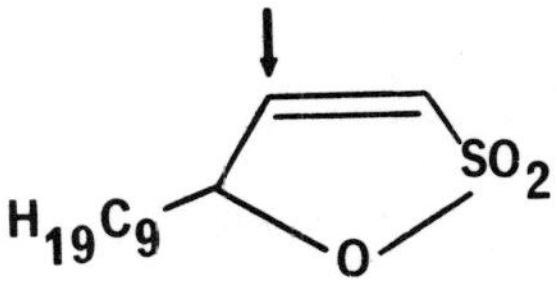

1-dodecene-1,3-sultone

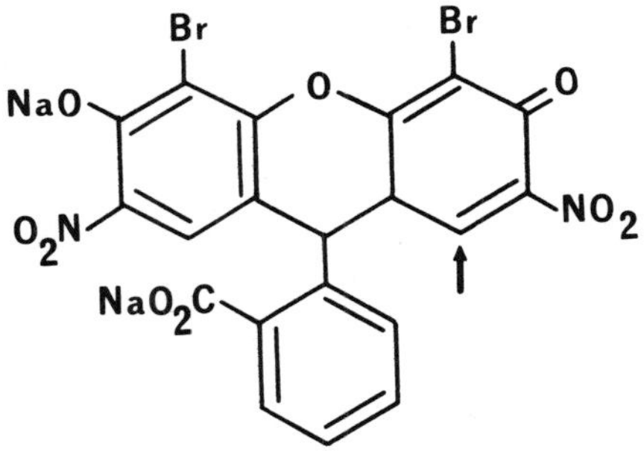

eosin

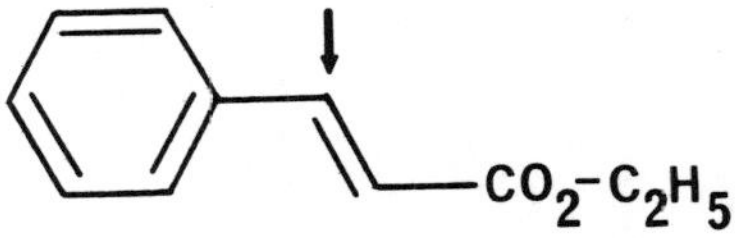

ethyl cinnamate

H CHO

formaldehyde

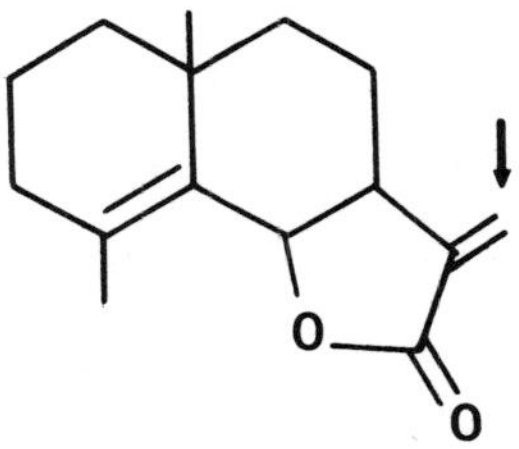

frullanolide

(continued)

Table 6   (continued)

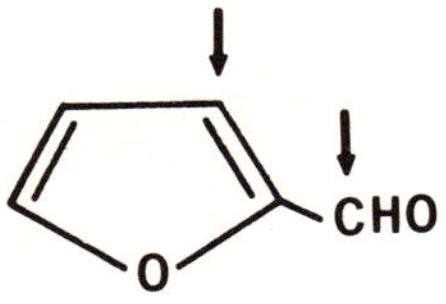

furfural

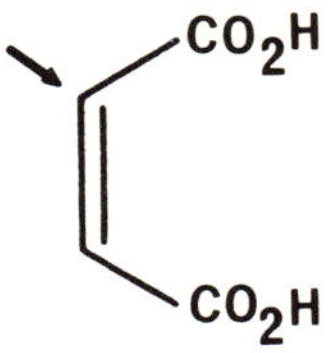

maleic acid

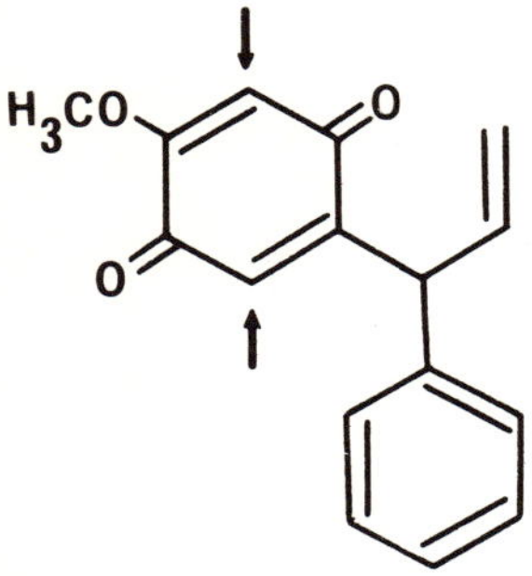

4-methoxydalbergione

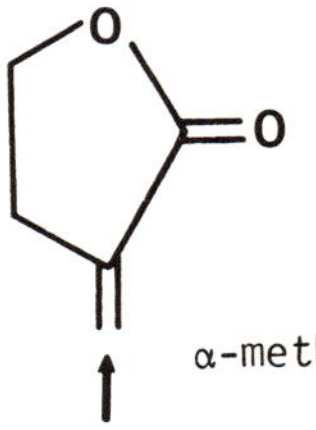

α-methylene-γ-butyrolactone
(tulipalin A)

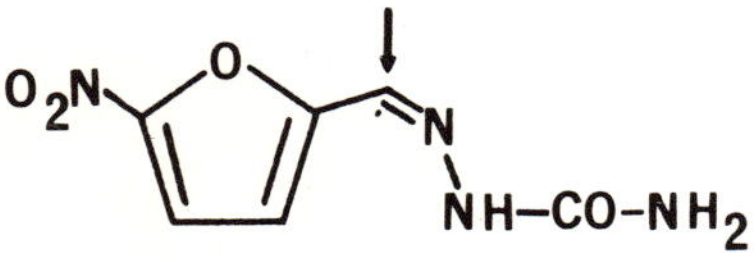

nitrofurazone

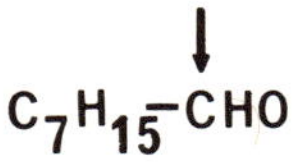

$C_7H_{15}-CHO$

octanaldehyde

(continued)

Table 6 (continued)

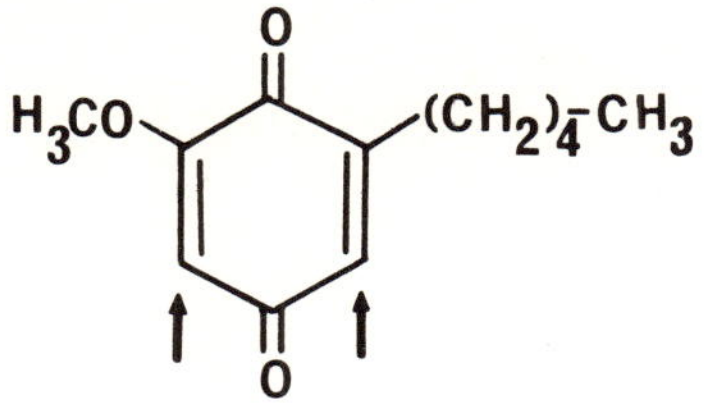

primine

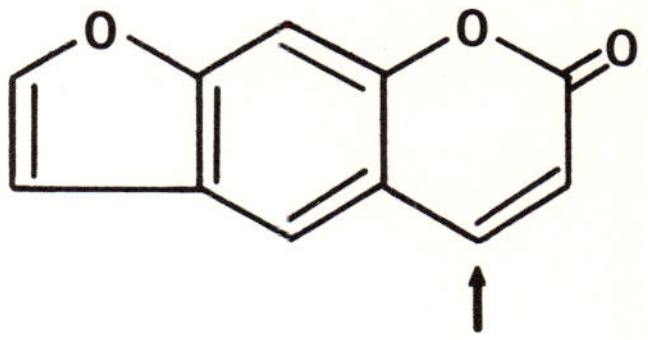

psoralen

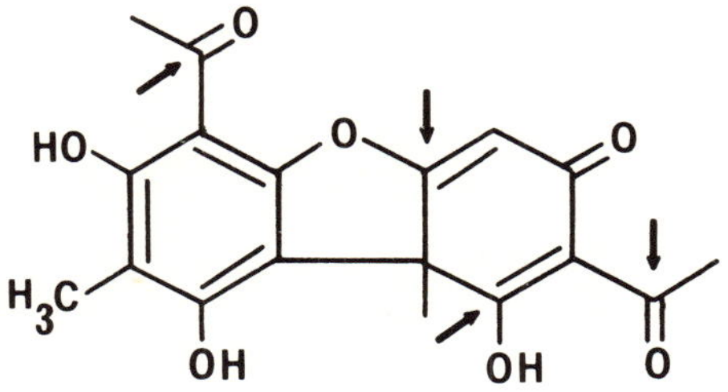

usnic acid

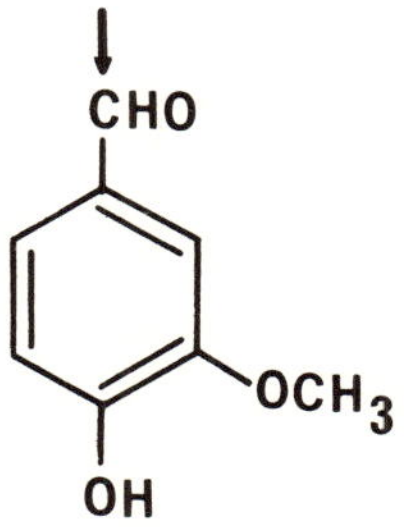

vanillin

Table 7 Haptens Susceptible to Radical Formation (loss of halogen)

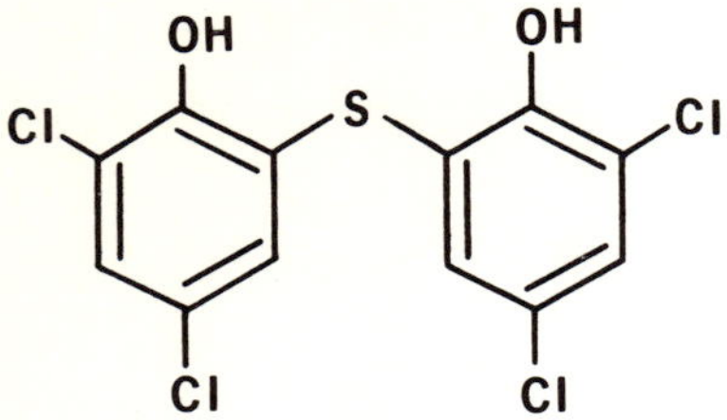

bithionol

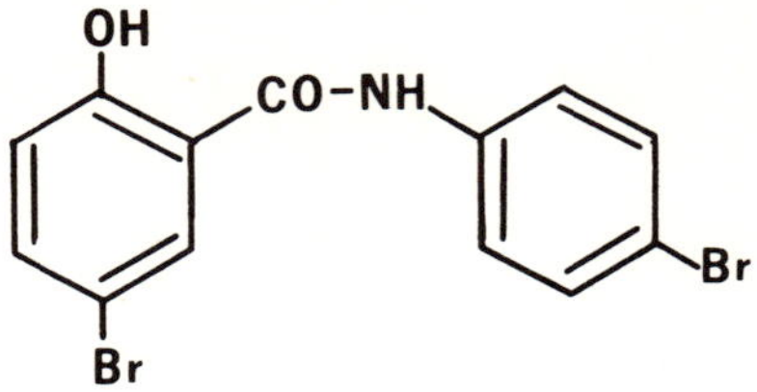

dibromosalicylanilide

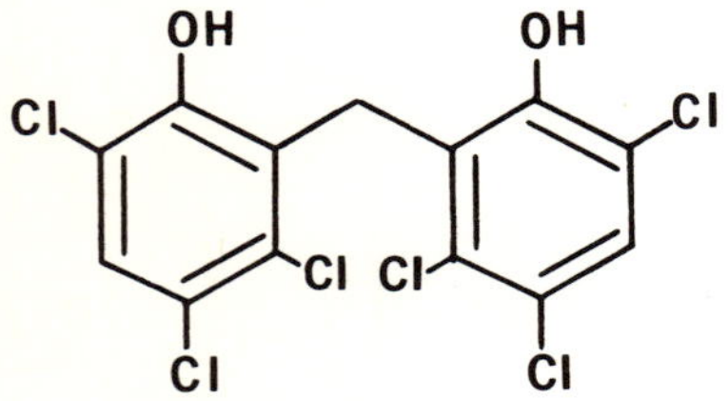

hexachlorophene

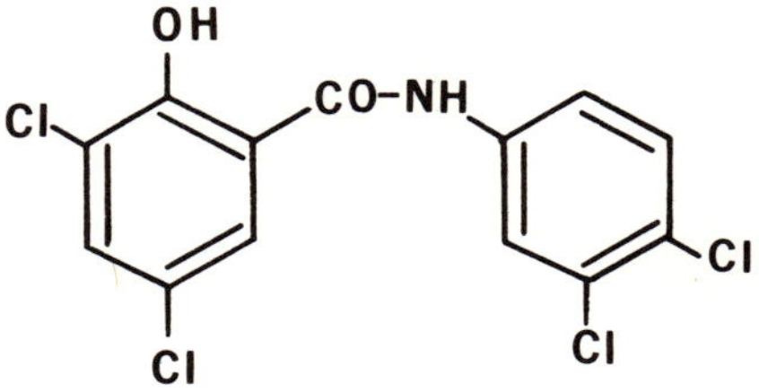

tetrachlorosalicylanilide

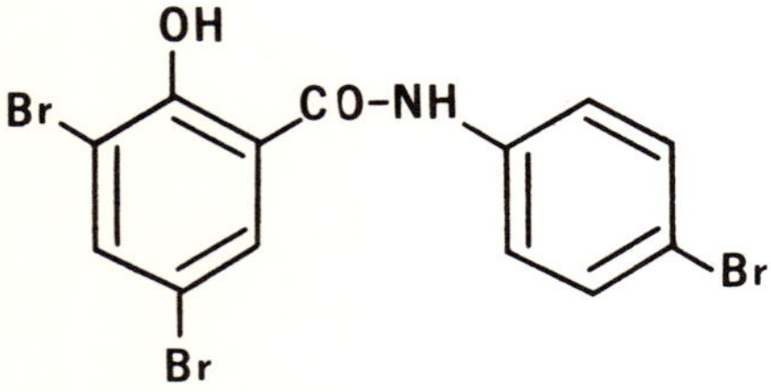

tribromosalicylanilide

Table 8 Haptens Susceptible to Nucleophilic Reactions
⟶: nucleophilic substitution, ⟶▷: nucleophilic addition

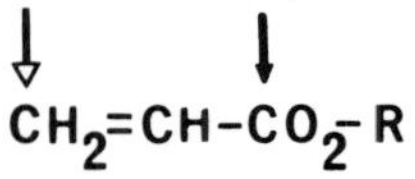

$CH_2=CH-CO_2-R$

acrylates

$Cl_3C-CH-OH$
          $|$
          OH

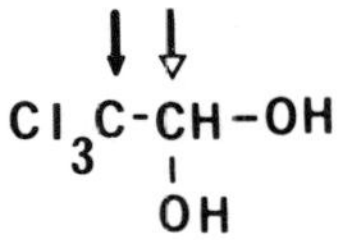

chloral hydrate

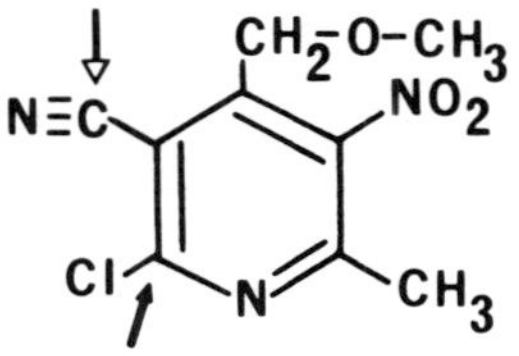

6-chloro-5-cyano-2-methyl-4-methoxymethyl-
3-nitropyridine

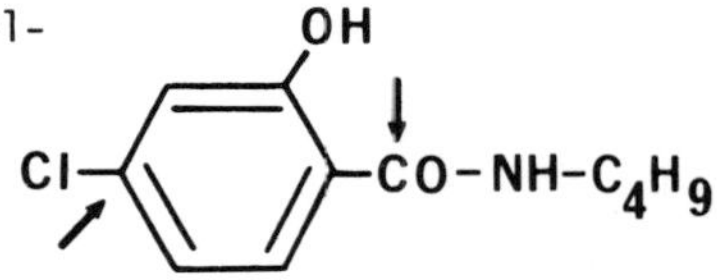

4-chloro-2-hydroxybenzoid acid
butylamide

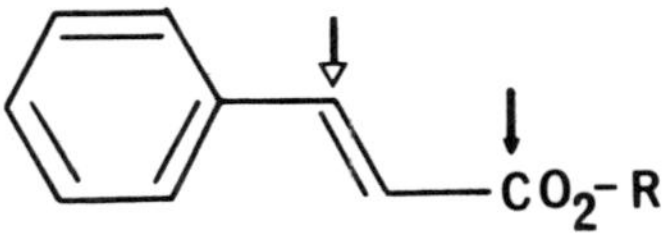

$R = C_2H_5$, ethyl cinnamate

$R = CH_2-C_6H_5$, benzyl cinnamate

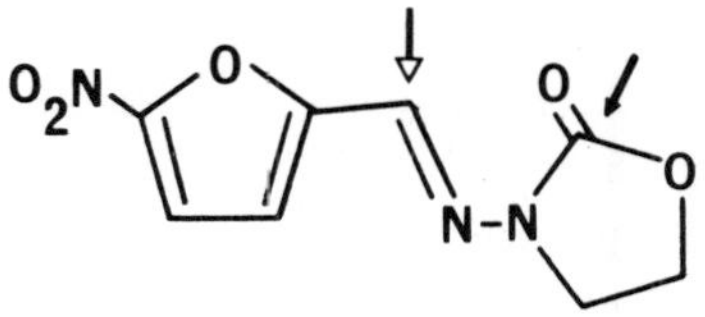

nitrofurazolidone

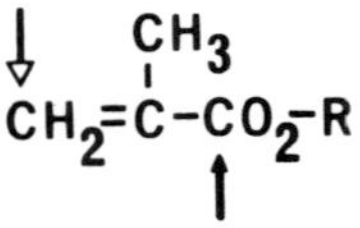

methacrylates

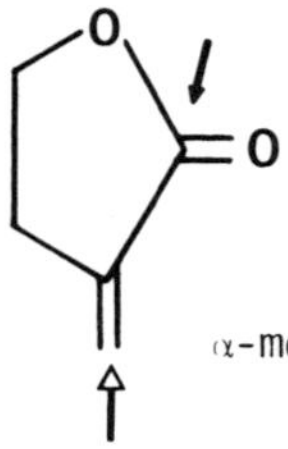

α-methylene-γ-butyrolactone

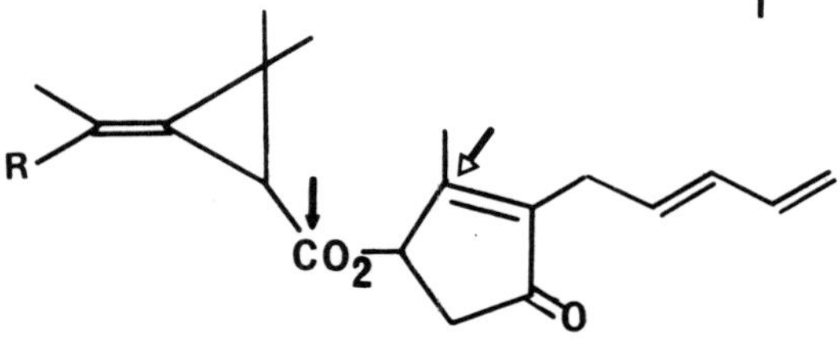

$R = CH_3$, pyrethrin I

$R = CO_2CH_3$, pyrethrin II

Table 9 Metal Salts Possessing Chelating Properties

Salt	Examples
Chromium	$K_2Cr_2O_7$, cement
Cobalt	$CoCl_6$, vitamin B_{12}, cement $Co_2(SO_4)_3$
Copper	$CuSO_4$
Gold	$AuCl_3$
Iron	$FeCl_3$
Manganese	$MnCl_2$
Mercury	$MgCl_2$, amalgams, merthiolate
Platinum	H_2PtCl_6

Prohaptens: The Concept of Prohapten

Not all haptens can react directly with a protein. Several of them need first to
undergo a chemical (or photochemical) transformation to become "reactive."
We shall refer to these chemicals as prohaptens.

The concept of prohapten is best illustrated in photoallergic reactions. If
a test with a hapten such as psoralen is carried out in the absence of light, no
positive reaction is observed (Herman and Sams, 1972). Activation (transformation) of the substance(s) by light irradiation produces a positive reaction.
This phenomenon is due to the transformation of the prohapten into a hapten
and a subsequent stimulation of the immune system. We shall see further
that cross reactivities between molecules of apparently unrelated structures
can only be explained if there is formation of a common metabolite. For instance, the cross-allergy observed in the case of hydroquinone and paraphenyl-
enediamine (PPD) can be explained by the in vivo formation of benzoquinone.

Another example of prohapten formation is found in ACD to urushiol (poison ivy). It is proposed that the catechol derivative (urushiol) is oxidized to the orthoquinone compound, which is then able to react with proteins (Dupuis, 1979; Mason and Lada, 1954; Mason, 1955).

pentadecylcatechol

Protection of the vicinal hydroxyl functions by methylation (pentadecylveratrole) produces an inactive (skin test) compound (Baer et al., 1966, 1970).

pentadecylveratrole

The concept of prohapten is an extremely important one. Failure, enzymatically or chemically, to convert a prohapten into a hapten may explain, in certain patients, the absence of cross-reactivities (observed in other patients) between common compounds.

Some chemical structures of prohaptens are illustrated in Table 10.

Reactions of Haptens with Proteins

A classification of haptens according to their reactivity has just been proposed. Let us consider the reactions of haptens, based on their *functional groups*, with the amino acid side chains of proteins.

Acids

ACD to acids is not common, but sensitivity to toluic (Emmett and Suskind, 1973) and maleic acids (Schwartz et al., 1948) has been reported. Organic acids may form salt bridges (see Chap. 5) with proteins.

Table 10 Prohaptens: These Compounds Must Undergo Chemical Modification(s) before Becoming True Haptens

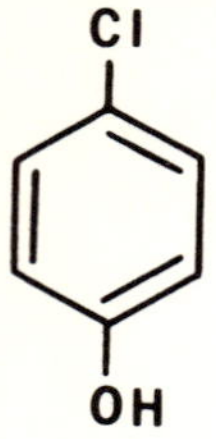

p-chlorophenol

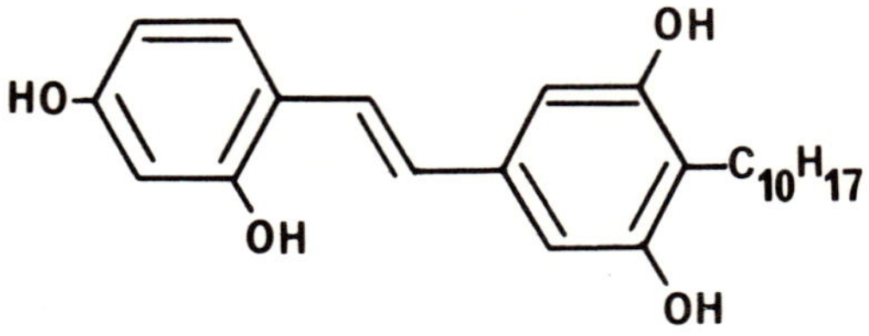

chlorophorin

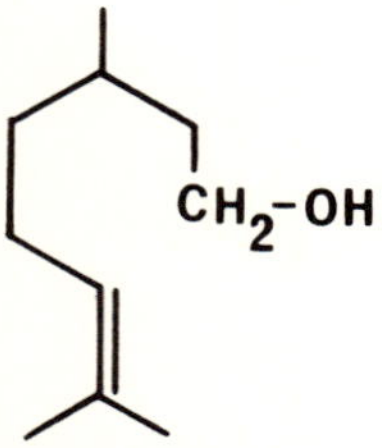

citronellol

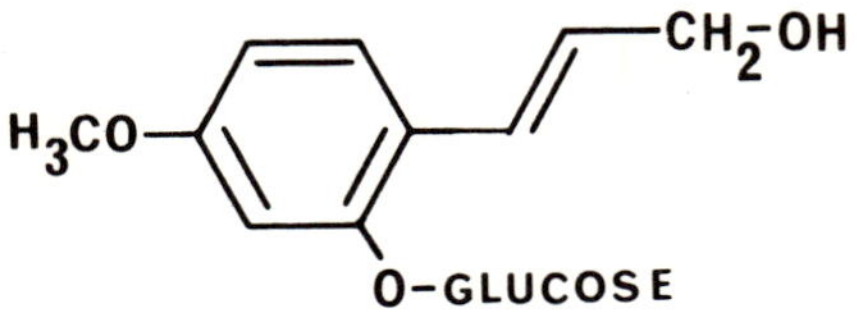

coniferin

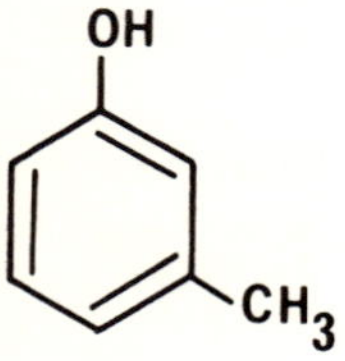

m-cresol

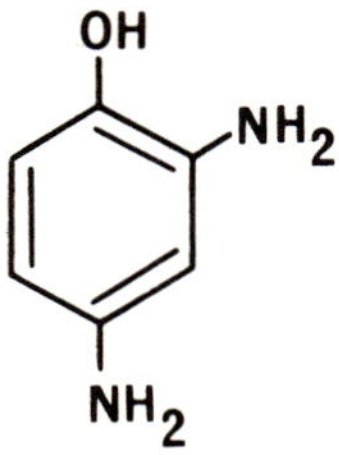

2,4-diaminophenol

(continued)

Table 10 (continued)

$HO-CH_2-CH_2-OH$

ethylene glycol

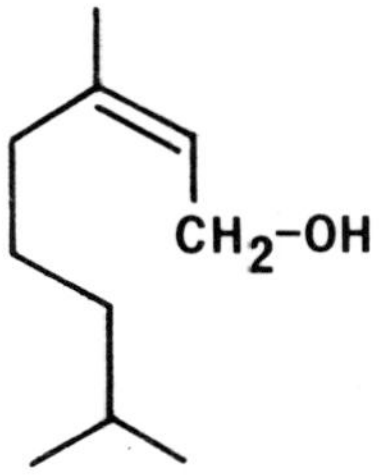

geraniol

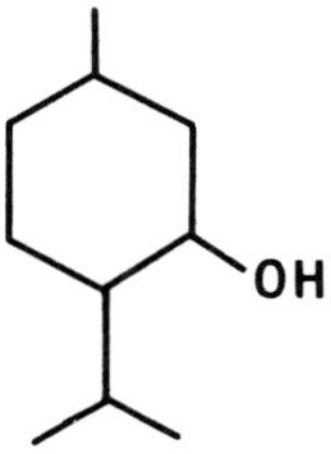

menthol

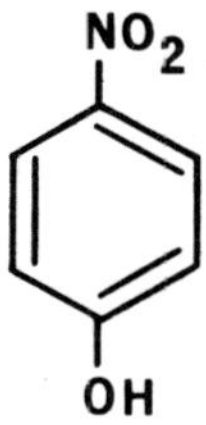

p-nitrophenol

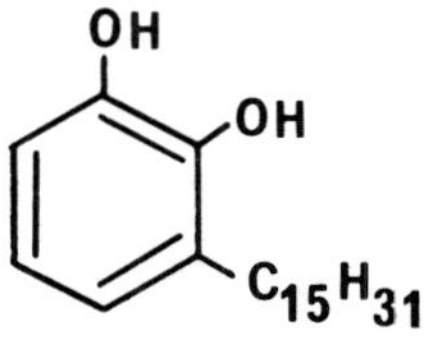

pentadecylcatechol

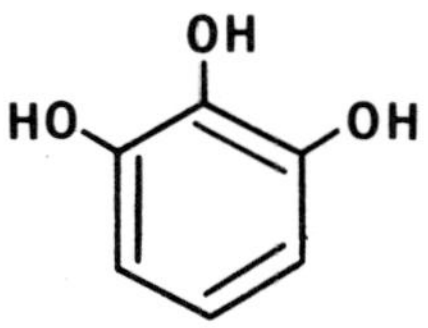

pyrogallol

(continued)

Table 10 (continued)

(a) Hydrocarbons → hydroperoxides

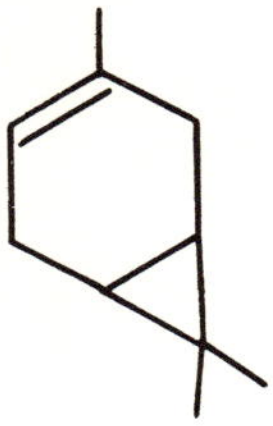

Δ^3-carene 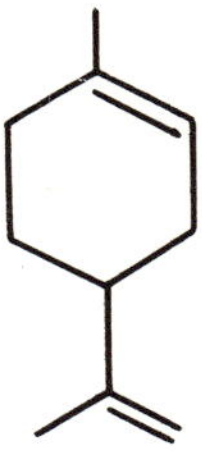   limonene 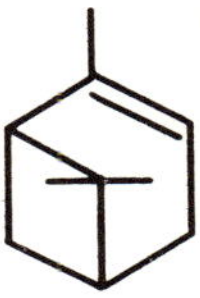   α-pinene

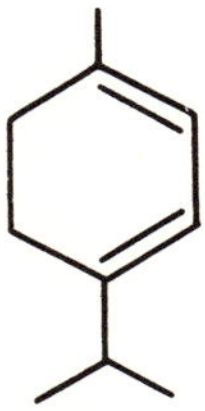

terpinene

(b) Alcohols or phenols → ketones (or aldehydes) or quinones

$H_2N-CH_2-CH_2-OH$

aminoethanol

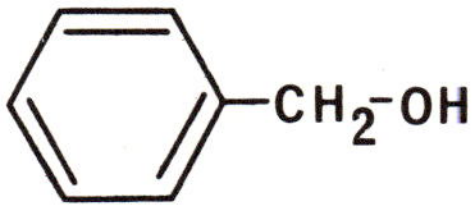

$-CH_2-OH$

benzyl alcohol

(continued)

Table 10 (continued)

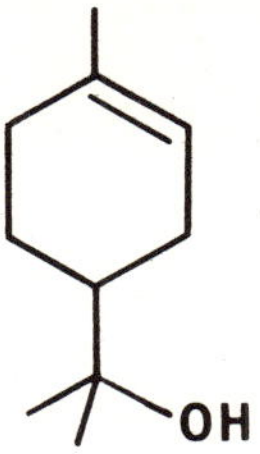

terpineol

<u>(c) Aromatic amines undergoing oxidation and/or hydrolysis</u>

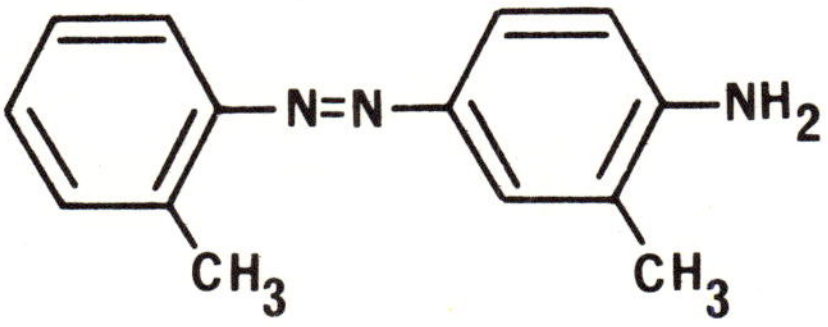

aminoazotoluene

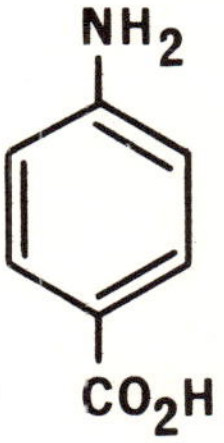

p-aminobenzoic acid

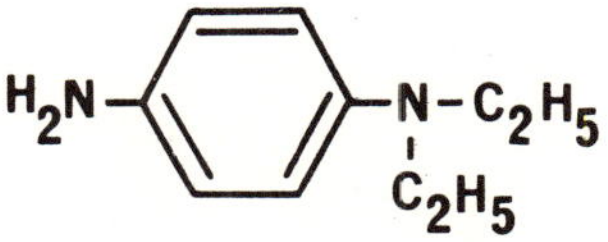

4-amino-N,N-diethylaniline

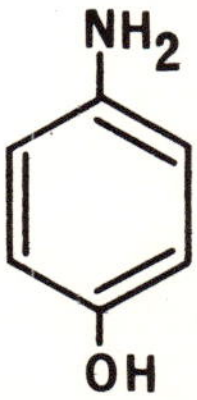

p-aminophenol

(continued)

Table 10 (continued)

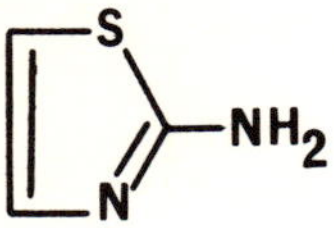

2-aminothiazole

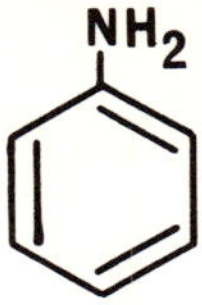

aniline

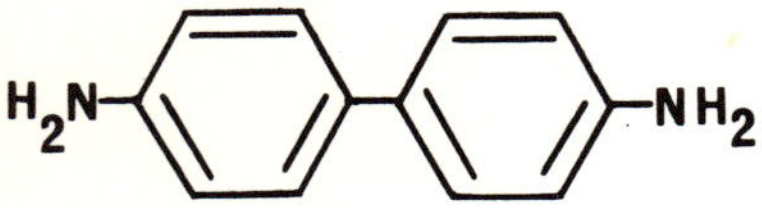

benzidine

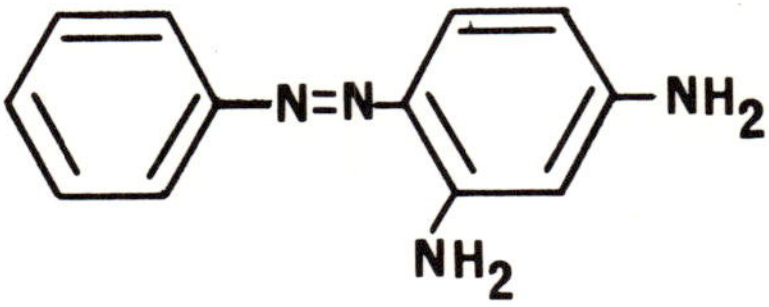

chrysoidin

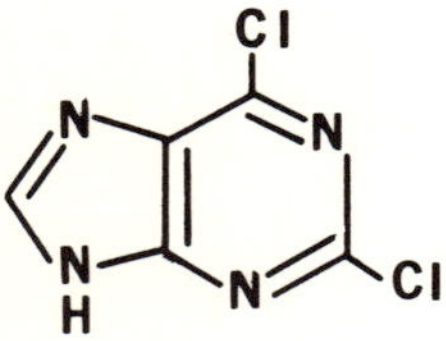

2,6-dichloropyrimidine

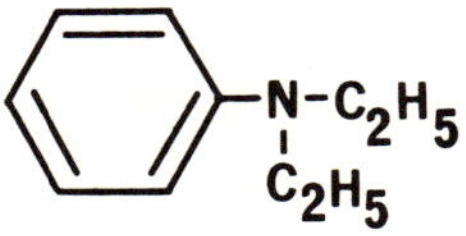

diethylaniline

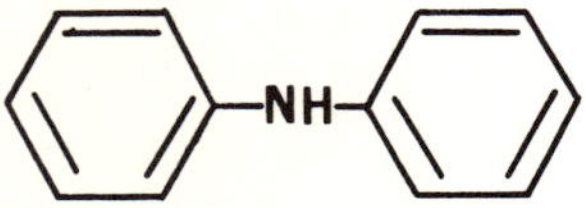

diphenylamine

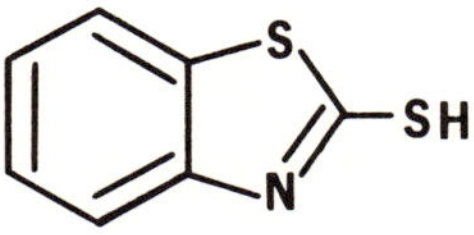

mercaptobenzothiazole

(continued)

Table 10   (continued)

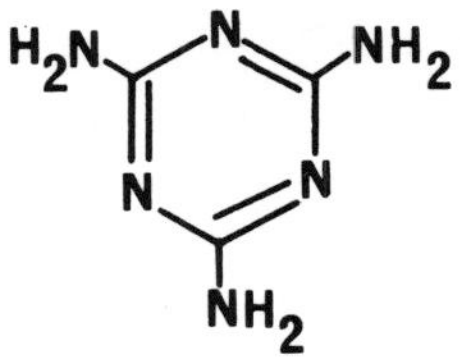

melamine

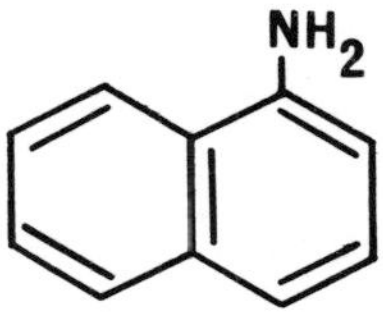

α-naphthylamine

d) miscellaneous

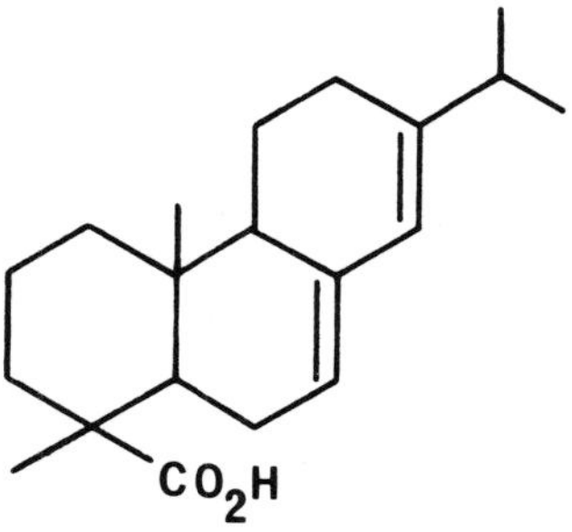

abietic acid

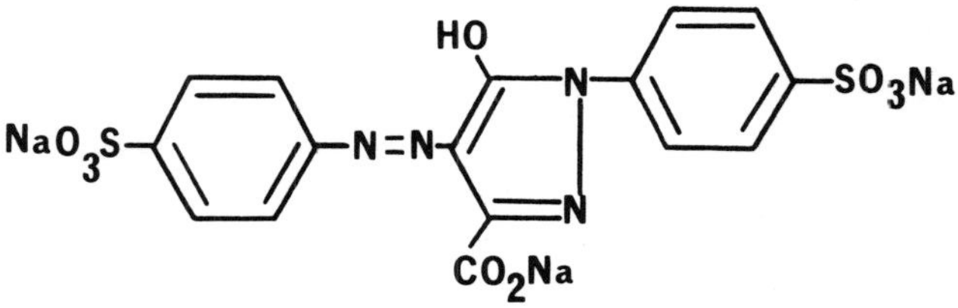

C. I. Acid Yellow 23

(continued)

Table 10 (continued)

$C_{16}H_{33}-\overset{+}{N}-(CH_3)_3$

cetavlon

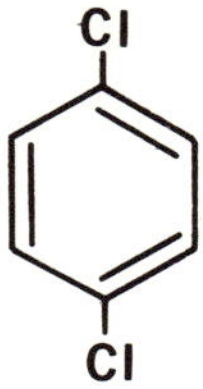

p-dichlorobenzene

$(HO-CH_2CH_2)_2-NH$

diethanolamine

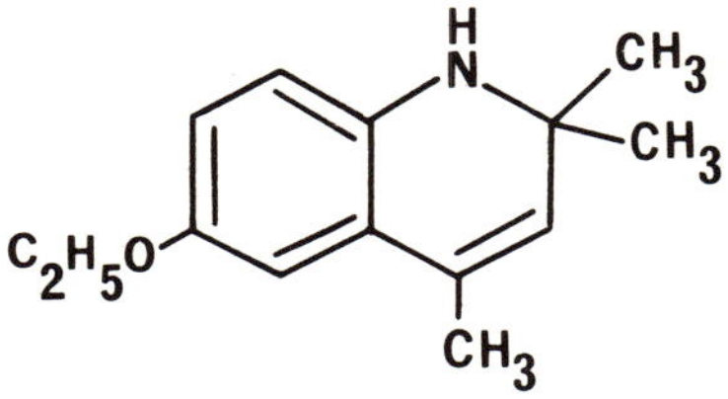

ethoxyquin

$H_2N-CH_2-CH_2-NH_2$

ethylenediamine

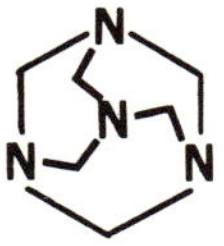

hexamethylenetetramine

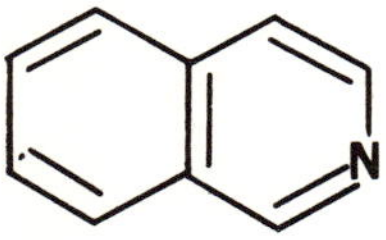

isoquinoline

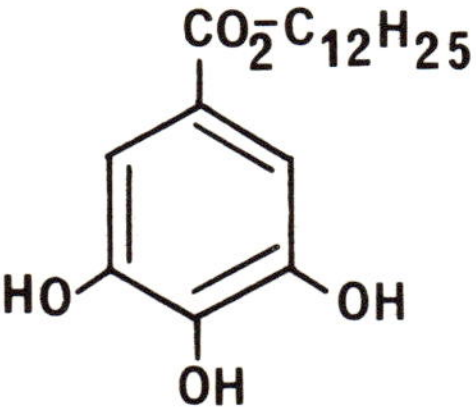

lauryl gallate

(continued)

Table 10 (continued)

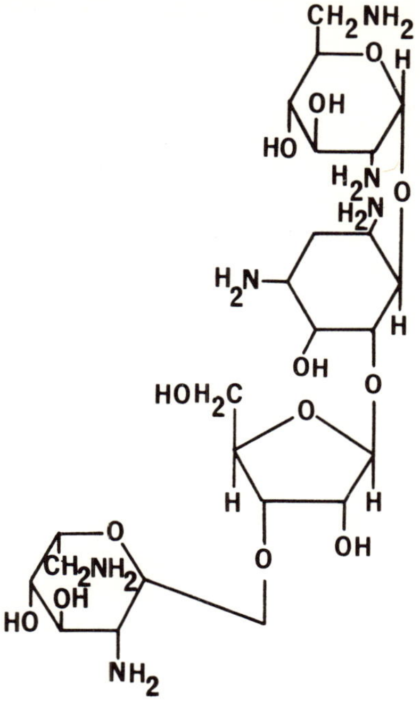

Neomycine

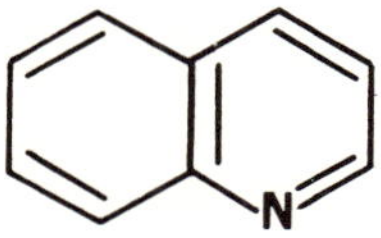

quinoline

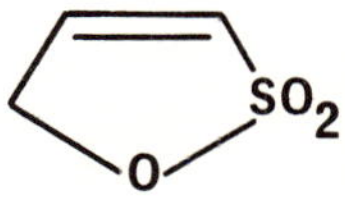

sultone

HS–CH$_2$–CO$_2$H

thioglycollic acid

N(CH$_2$–CH$_2$–OH)$_3$

triethanolamine

$$R-COO^- \quad\quad\quad\quad\quad\quad\quad\quad\quad\quad R-COO^-$$
$$\text{or} \quad + \quad NH_3^+\text{- protein} \longrightarrow \quad \text{or} \quad \Big\} \ NH_3^+\text{- protein}$$
$$R-SO_3^- \quad\quad\quad\quad\quad\quad\quad\quad\quad\quad R-SO_3^-$$

It is also conceivable that aromatic acids are decarboxylated and oxidized in vivo (to give phenols for instance and then quinones) and that aromatic sulfonic acids are transformed into phenols ($Ar-SO_3H \rightarrow ArOH$), a reaction that is known in chemistry. These oxidized species can be attacked by a nucleophilic amino acid side chain of the protein and become covalently bound.

Aldehydes

Contact allergy to aldehydes is well known and can involve such simple aldehydes as formaldehyde, a compound frequently used in the textile, plastic, and tanning industries. Allergy resulting from contact with naturally occurring aldehydes (vanillin, citral, citronellal, etc.) has also been reported (Foussereau and Benezra, 1970, 1982).

Aldehydes can readily form imines (Schiff bases) with primary or secondary amines or react with alcohols to form hemiacetals.

$$R-C{\overset{O}{\underset{H}{}}} \quad + \quad NH_3^+\text{-protein} \longrightarrow R-CH=NH^+\text{-protein}$$

(an imine)

$$R-C{\overset{O}{\underset{H}{}}} \quad + \quad HO\text{-protein} \longrightarrow R-\underset{OH}{CH}-O\text{-protein}$$

(a hemiacetal)

$$H-C{\overset{O}{\underset{H}{}}} \quad + \quad NH_3^+\text{-protein} \longrightarrow HO-CH_2-NH_2^+\text{-protein}$$

formaldehyde

It is known that naturally occurring aldehydes, such as pyridoxal phosphate (vitamin B_6), do form a reversible Schiff base with the ϵ-amino group of lysine at the active site of decarboxylases and transaminases (Jenkins and Sizer, 1959). Schiff base formation is probably the mechanism by which aldehydes combine with a carrier.

Amines

Some amines are among the most common allergens. For instance, Fisher (1973) mentions that PPD and ethylenediamine are the most frequent causative agents of ACD among his patients. Amines are used in plastic and rubber industries, in creams and ointments, in dyes, resins, leather processing, etc.

In the case of primary amines, it is unlikely that such compounds interact directly with protein carrier(s), although they can form salt bridges. There has been a report of this type of interaction between DNP-poly-L-lysine conjugate and proteins (Green et al., 1966). Primary amines are more likely to be oxidized in vivo (by monoamine oxidase) to aldehydes (or acids) prior to their reaction with a carrier.

$$R-CH_2-NH_2 \xrightarrow{[O]} R-CH=NH \xrightarrow{H_2O} R-CHO$$

Aromatic amines (unsubstituted and N-alkylated) are probably oxidized to the corresponding quinones as suggested by Mayer (1930). Quinones, in turn, are electrophilic systems and can undergo nucleophilic additions (see Chap. 5).

Quaternary ammonium salts are rare and inconsistent sensitizers (Foussereau and Benezra, 1970, 1982; Huriez et al., 1965). These compounds are commonly used in antiseptic detergents. They may be illustrative examples of electrostatic interactions with the carrier or, alternately, they may be oxidized in vivo to yield aldehydes.

Diazo Compounds

These compounds are used as dyes. They are composed of many substituted aromatic nuclei and, according to the degree of conjugation, form compounds with an intense absorption in the visible spectrum. The following structures illustrate some diazo compounds.

C. I. Direct Red 28 (Congo red)

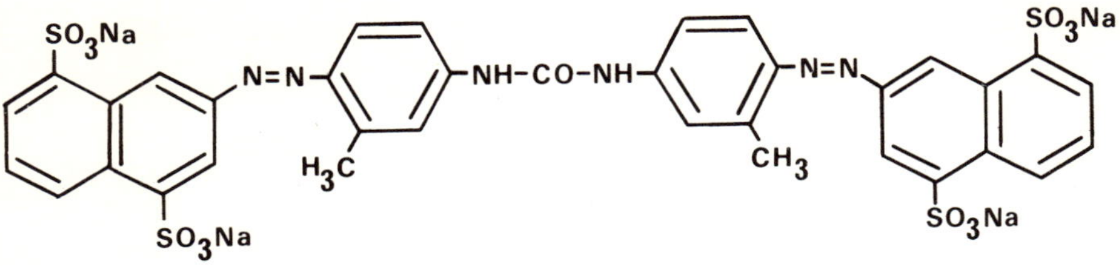

C. I. Direct Yellow 50

These compounds are probably not stable in vivo and may be cleaved to give aromatic amines of the PPD type, which can then be converted to quinones.

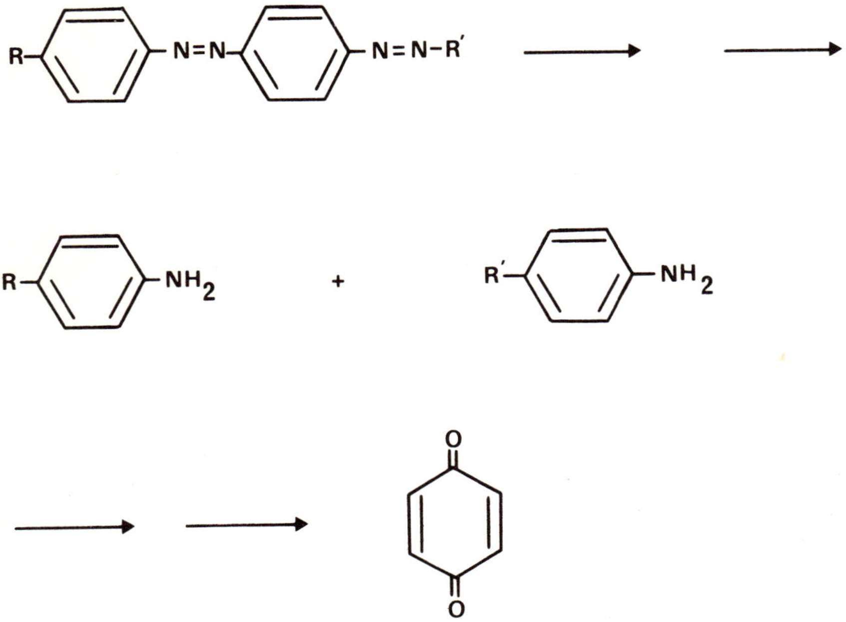

Esters

Esters are usually easily hydrolyzable to the corresponding alcohol and acid, which can then be metabolized further to give reactive compounds. Benzocaine, a compound used in many topical anesthetics, is a potent sensitizer (Foussereau and Benezra, 1970, 1982). It can by hydrolyzed to p-aminobenzoic

acid and ethanol. It is probable that the amino acid is further oxidized to
the corresponding *p*-quinone.

Esters can also undergo transesterification and alcohol-amine interchanges.
For instance, reaction of benzocaine with lysine residues will yield *p*-amino-
benzoyllysyl protein, a stable derivative.

Ethers

Aliphatic ethers are stable compounds and are not easily cleaved at the carbon-
oxygen bond. Cleavage can be accomplished chemically, however, with the
use of strong acids, such as HI, or Lewis acids, such as $AlCl_3$, and heat (Fieser
and Fieser, 1967). Highly substituted ethers are more easily cleaved because
cleavage results in a release of steric hindrance. Reported sensitivity to ethers
may be due to other chemicals present in these commercial preparations or to
the formation of autooxidation products such as hydroperoxides.
    Phenolic ethers are, however, much less stable than aliphatic ethers and de-
compose to give phenol and alkyl (or aryl) moieties. For instance, methyl
ethers of substituted phenols can yield, by the action of methyl transferases,
a phenol residue that can be further oxidized to a quinone derivative.

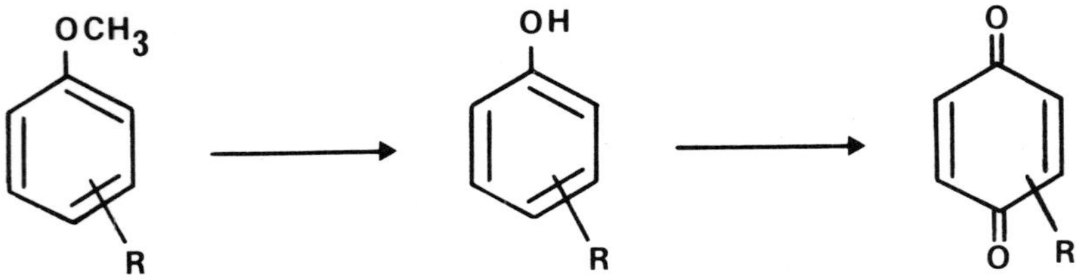

The stability of these ethers depends also on the facility of removal of the alkyl (or aryl) group. For instance, benzyl ether can be cleaved easily, as illustrated in the case of contact allergy to hydroquinone monobenzylether, a depigmenting agent also used as rubber antioxidant (Sidi et al., 1964).

Substituted catechol derivatives also fall into this category. In particular, dimethoxycatechols can yield *o*- or *p*-quinones by the action of catechol o-methyl transferase and phenolases (Mason and Lada, 1954; Mason, 1955). Nevertheless protection of hydroxyl groups in pentadecyl catechol by methylation ($-OCH_3$) results in a largely diminished allergic activity (Baer et al., 1966; 1970).

Epoxides

Epoxides are very reactive compounds that can undergo base-catalyzed or acid-catalyzed opening. They can readily undergo nucleophilic attack by the ϵ-amino group of lysine residues. Strictly speaking, the reaction can occur at the *a* or *b* positions as illustrated by the following equations.

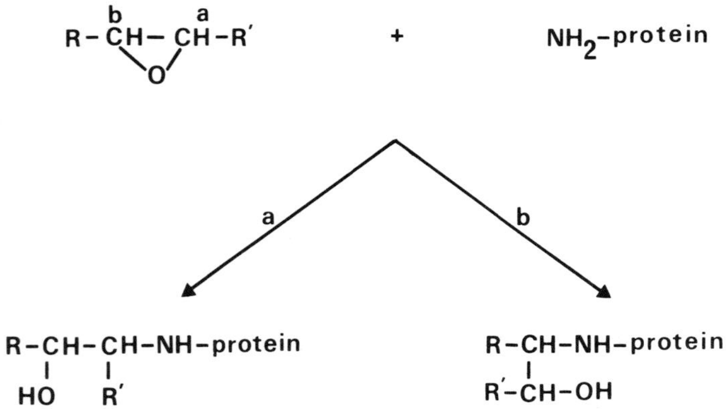

The direction of opening will be governed by factors such as the nature of the nucleophile, the degree of substitution of the epoxides, the conditions of reactions, etc. These factors are not probably very important in the case of adduct formation related to ACD. More relevant, however, is the relative ease with which the epoxide can be opened. The facility of ring opening is related to the structure of the epoxide. The nucleophilic attack (Reeve and Sadle, 1950) will occur at the less substituted carbon atom.

ACD to epoxides is generally encountered in allergy to resins: since epoxy resins usually contain epoxides of the type CH_2-CH-R, the compounds will react with proteins to form the corresponding conjugates because of small steric hindrance.

Halogenated Compounds

The ease of nucleophilic displacement of aliphatic halides is extremely variable. Primary halides $R-CH_2-X$ are more easily substituted than secondary (RR'-CHX) or tertiary (RRR'CX) halides. Primary carbons bearing a chlorine atom can undergo nucleophilic attack readily if they are part of a chloromethyl-ketone system.

$$Tos-NH-Lys-\overset{\displaystyle O}{\overset{\|}{C}}_{\diagdown CH_2-Cl}$$

```
tosyllysinechloromethylketone (TLCK)
```

This particular system is the basis of irreversible inhibition of trypsin and chymotrypsin by tosyllysinechloromethylketone (TLCK) (Shaw et al., 1965) and by tosylphenylalaninechloromethylketone (TPCK) (Ong et al., 1965; Schoellman and Shaw, 1963), respectively. Such a system is present in known haptens, the fungicide clophenoxide, and ω-chloroacetophenone (Foussereau and Benezra, 1970, 1982). The particular reactivity of the halogen is due, in the case of these compounds, to the electron-withdrawing effect of the keto function with the net result of a decrease in the electronic density of the chloro-substituted carbon.

Halogenated aromatic compounds undergo nucleophilic substitution less easily than aliphatic halides. This is because the aromatic nucleus is electron-rich and shows no tendency to further attack by a nucleophile (i.e., another electron-rich species). However, when there are electron-withdrawing groups (such as NO_2, CN, $COCH_3$, etc) *ortho* or *para* to the halogen, nucleophilic substitution becomes easy: the aromatic nucleus is now electron deficient and electron-rich species can attack it. The negative charge appearing on the nucleus is "absorbed" by the electron withdrawing groups, as in the following example.

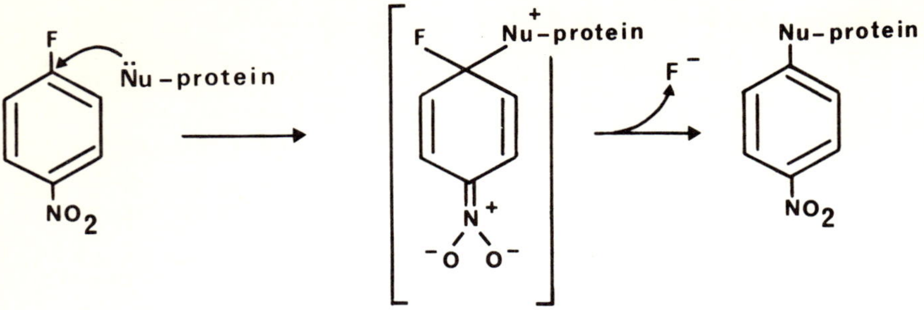

This may explain the extraordinary sensitizing capacity of DNCB, DNFB, and picryl chloride: the more electron-withdrawing groups on the nucleus, the more reactive is the halogen.

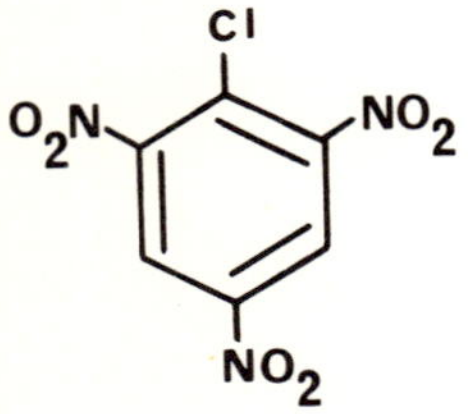

picryl chloride

Substituted halogenated aromatic compounds such as DDT, chloropromazine, hexachlorophene, TCSA, etc., which are all strong allergens, can react with proteins either by nucleophilic attack or, more likely by free radical formation.

Quinones

Allergy to quinones is well documented (Foussereau et al., 1969; Foussereau and Benezra, 1970, 1982; Mayer, 1950). These compounds are used in commercial preparations such as plastics, rubber, cosmetics, etc. They can occur naturally in plants, such as primin in *Primula obconica* (Fregert et al., 1968; Hausen, 1973). Quinones possess an electrophilic system that can undergo a Michael-type addition with a suitable nucleophile, forming adducts. The in vitro demonstration of this mechanism has been reported for the coupling of *o*-pentadecylquinone to human serum albumin (HSA) (Mason and Lada, 1954) and bovine gammaglobulin (BGG) (Byck and Dawson, 1968) and for the reaction of oxidized urushiol with HSA and human skin proteins (Dupuis, 1979). These adducts have been shown to possess immunological properties (Dupuis, 1979; Mason and Lada, 1954).

Salts from Metals

ACD to salts from metals is frequent. Very often it involves allergy to mercuric salts (Morris, 1960; Taugner and Schültz, 1966), chromate ions (Jaeger and Pelloni, 1950; Johnston and Calnan, 1958; Pirilä, 1954; Polak and Frey, 1973; Thulin and Zacharinae, 1972), cobalt salts (Delacretaz and Geiser, 1960; Salinas and Subiza, 1956), and nickel salts (Fisher, 1973). Only two cases of allergy to iron have been reported (Baer, 1973).

It is not clear how these metallic salts can induce sensitization or provoke cutaneous reactions. One property shared by these metals is that they are transition metals and are prone to form complexes. These metals posses a co-ordination number ranging from 4 to 6 due to unfilled orbitals (Storck and Schwarz, 1960). Complexes of some of these metals are known to occur in biological systems.

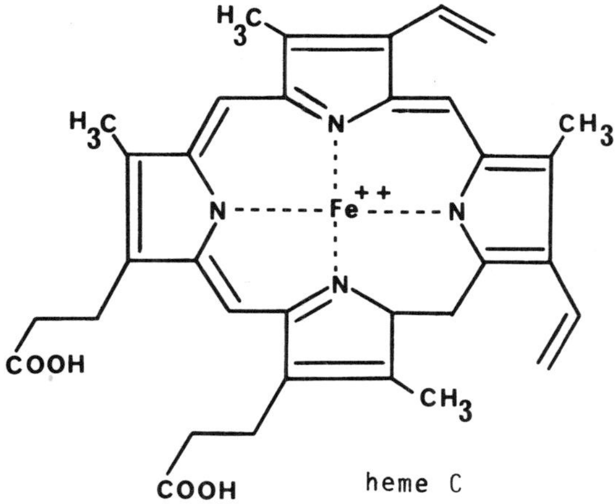

It is probable that these metals combine with suitable protein and form complexes, which result in conformational changes. Since it is known that conformational changes in proteins greatly influence their antigenic properties (Atassi, 1975; St-Rose and Cinader, 1967), this can explain why metallic salts are allergenic. In this connection, it is tempting to postulate that niobium and vanadium salts, for instance, should be sensitizers. However, exposure to these metals is rare, explaining why such allergies have not been reported so far. Metals that do not form complexes (e.g., Na$^+$, K$^+$, Li$^+$) have not been reported as causative agents of ACD.

The nature of the amino acids important for complex formation (in proteins) with transition metals has not been investigated. Electron donors from side-chain residues, such as cysteine, methionine, histidine, lysine, etc., can be expected to participate in complex formation. The oxygen of the carbonyl function and the amino group of the peptide bond may also play a role in the coordination process. Water molecules may be involved in salt-protein complexes. In vitro studies of ACD to salts have been performed with metal salts alone (Gross et al., 1968), in combination with albumin (Mirza et al., 1974), or with amino acids (Hutchison et al., 1975; Shmunes et al., 1973).

Unsaturated Compounds

Monosaturated compounds are known to form peroxides by exposure to air (Hellerström et al., 1963). The peroxides can undergo reactions·with suitable nucleophiles and form adducts.

In this connection, it has been proposed that ACD to aged turpentine is caused by oxidation of Δ^3-carene (Hellerström et al., 1963):

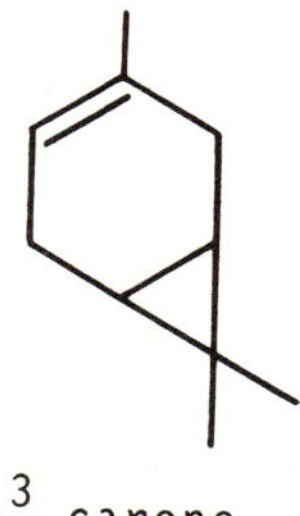

Freshly distilled (unoxidized) turpentine does not give a positive patch test in patients sensitive to turpentine.

The position α to a double bond also is susceptible to oxidation (allylic oxidation) and this results in hydroperoxide formation. The well-known oxidation of cholesterol illustrates this point (Van Lier and Smith, 1970).

cholesterol

Hydroperoxides can form radicals and react with proteins.

$$R-O-OH \longrightarrow R-O^{\bullet} + HO^{\bullet}$$

Polyunsaturated conjugated compounds can also readily form peroxides. The action of heat or light on these substances will produce ionic or radical species, which are exceptionally reactive. ACD to carotenes (Seidmann, 1946; Vickers, 1941) and to vitamin A (used in cosmetics) (Fisher, 1973) may be explained in this way.

Contact with aromatic hydrocarbons (anthracene, pyrene, etc.) contained in coal tar used in shampoos, creams, lotions, ointments, etc., usually results, in sensitive subjects, in a photoallergic reaction rather than a simple ACD.

7
Cross-Sensitization

The term "cross-sensitization" is used to denote the phenomenon where an allergic sensitization engendered by one compound extends to one or more other compounds (Baer, 1954). The allergen causing the primary reaction is referred to as the primary sensitizer or allergen. Secondary allergens are compounds that can cause cross-sensitization and are, in general, chemically related to the primary allergen.

Immunochemical Relationships between Primary and Secondary Allergens

The possible immunochemical relationships between primary and secondary allergens have been discussed by Baer (1954) and are reproduced here with modifications.

1. Structure similarities between primary and secondary allergens are so close that the immune system reacts against each one as if they were identical.
2. The primary allergen is converted in vivo into a compound that is either identical with the secondary allergen or so closely related to it that sensitized cells do not differentiate between them.
3. The secondary allergen may be transformed in vivo into compounds closely related to the primary allergen. In this case, the immunological system will be stimulated equally well by either compound.

4. Both primary and secondary allergens are converted in vivo into identical
    or very closely related chemicals.

An additional possibility has to be considered. Haptens have to be regarded
not only as isolated molecules, but as a part of a hapten-carrier complex. In
allergic contact dermatitis (ACD) to simple chemicals, it has been established
that hapten recognition is accomplished by antibodies directed against the
hapten, whereas carrier recognition is mainly due to a cellular phenomenon
(see Chap. 1). Some antibodies can, however, be directed against the carrier.
Thus, if one considers the hapten-carrier complex, a fifth possibility has to be
added to Baer's list:

5. Primary and secondary allergens combine with a carrier in vivo and are
    subsequently modified to form an antigen with similar determinants.

The Role of Simple Chemicals in Cross-Sensitization

Systematic studies of cross-sensitization were done initially at the beginning
of this century (Bloch, 1911). They involved cross-sensitization between iodoform and iodinated or methylated compounds. This work was followed by
investigations of cross-sensitization in hypersensitivity to quinine, formalin,
and resorcinol (Bloch, 1924).

These early studies were followed by the work of other investigators, which
resulted in the establishment of a critical role for chemical function similarities in cross-sensitization. The following is a discussion of some well-estab-
lished cross-sensitization to specific chemicals. In addition, Table 1 illustrates
cases of cross-sensitization among haptens of well-defined chemical structure.

Halogenated Hydroxyquinolines

Cross-sensitization between substituted 8-hydroxyquinolines has been reported
(Leifer and Steiner, 1951). Patients became sensitive to Diiodoquin (5,7-diiodo-
8-hydroxyquinoline) or to Vioform (5-chloro-7-iodo-8-hydroxyquinoline).
These patients showed cross-reaction to other 8-hydroxyquinoline derivatives,
but did not give a positive response to halogenated quinolines or quinoline
alone (Table 2, Fig. 1).

These observations pointed out the importance of the hydroxyl function
in position 8 of the quinoline structure and suggested that the true allergen,
i.e., the primary allergen was not the 8-hydroxyquinoline derivative, but some
other degradation product. This suggestion was elegantly confirmed when

Table 1 Cross-Reactivity between Some Common Chemicals

Compound	Uses	Cross-reactant

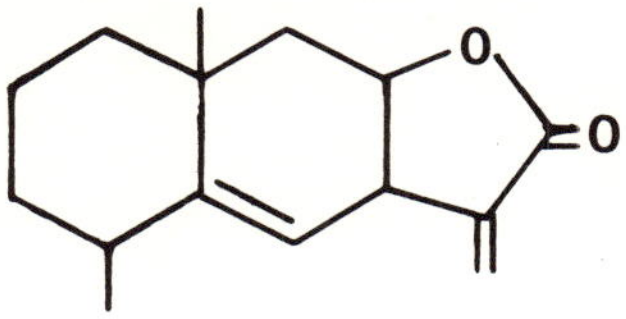

alantolactone — anthelminthic agent, naturally occurring — frullanolide

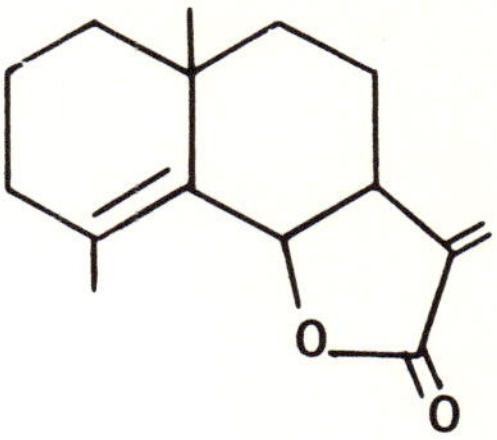

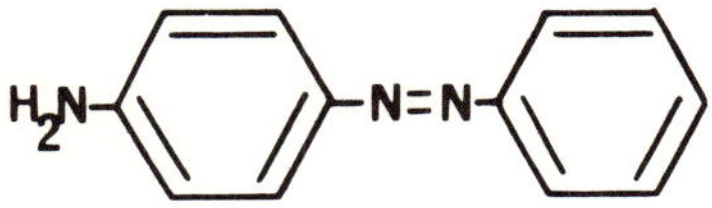

p-aminoazobenzene — leather dye — H_2N—R (p-amino compounds)

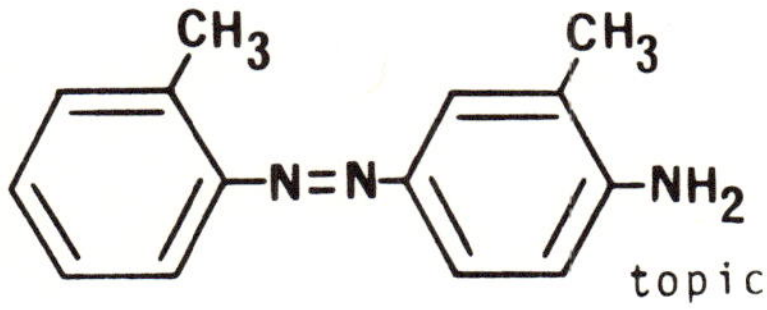

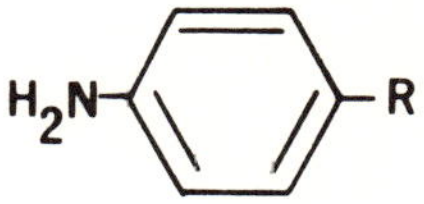

p-aminoazotoluene — topical medication — p-phenylenediamine (PPD)

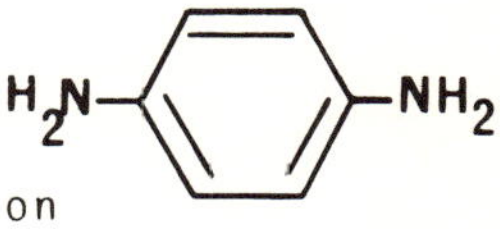

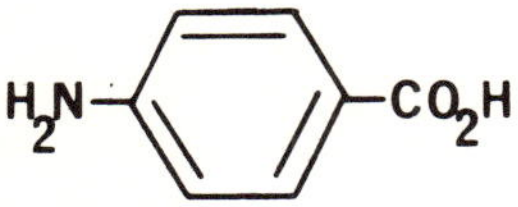

p-aminobenzoic acid — naturally occurring — p-phenylenediamine (PPD)

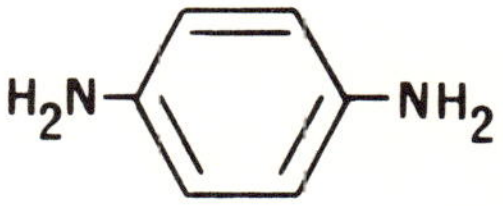

aniline — dyes, inks — H_2N—R (p-amino compounds)

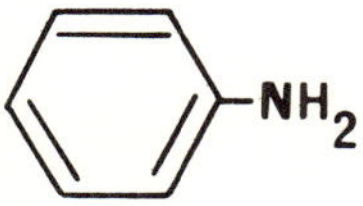

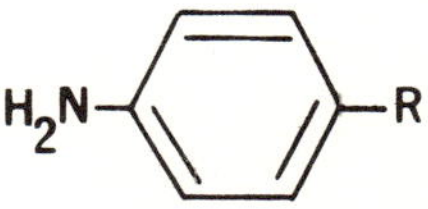

(continued)

Table 1 (continued)

Compound	Uses	Cross-reactant
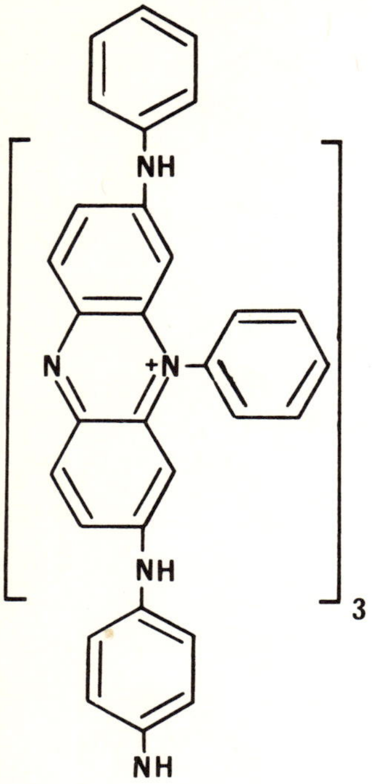 aniline black	fur dye	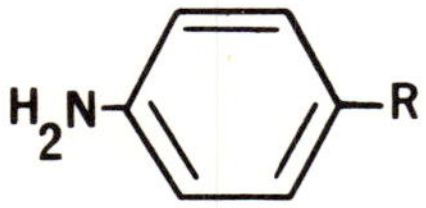 p-amino compounds
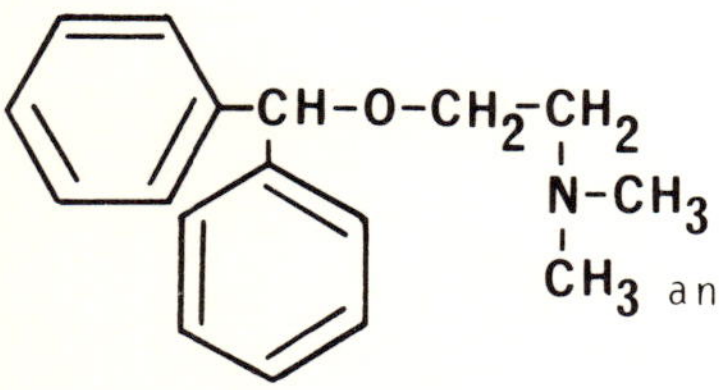 benadryl	antihistamine	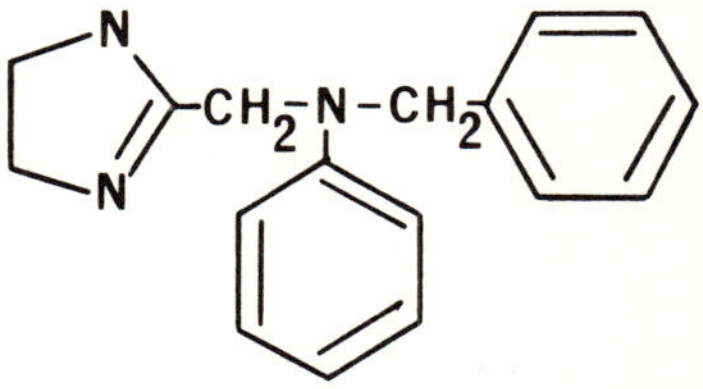 antistine

(continued)

Table 1 (continued)

Compound	Uses	Cross-reactant

benzaldehyde — $-CHO$

dyes, perfumery
naturally occurring

vanillin — CHO, OCH_3, OH

benzocain — H_2N- ... $-CO_2^-C_2H_5$

nesthetic

procain — H_2N- ... $-CO_2-CH_2CH_2-N-CH_3$, CH_3

benzoyl peroxide — $-CO_3H$

resins, ointments

ethyl benzoate — $-CO_2^-C_2H_5$

bismark brown — H_2N- ... $-N=N-$ ... $-N=N-$ ... H_2N, H_2N

dyes

p-amino compounds — H_2N- ... $-R$

(continued)

Table 1 (continued)

Compound	Uses	Cross-reactant

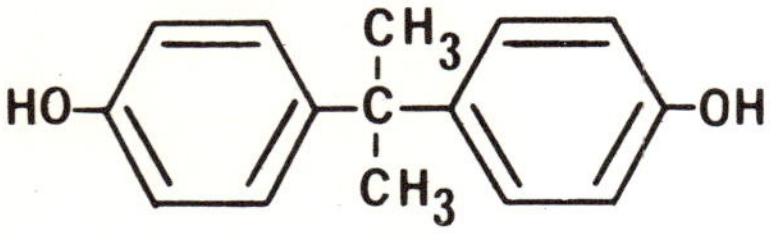

bisphenol A　　epoxy resins

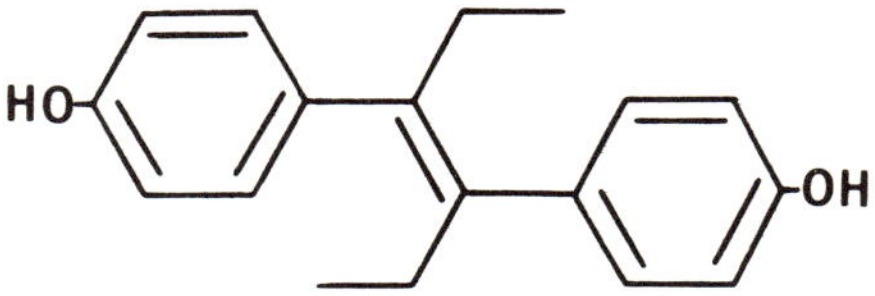

diethylstilbestrol

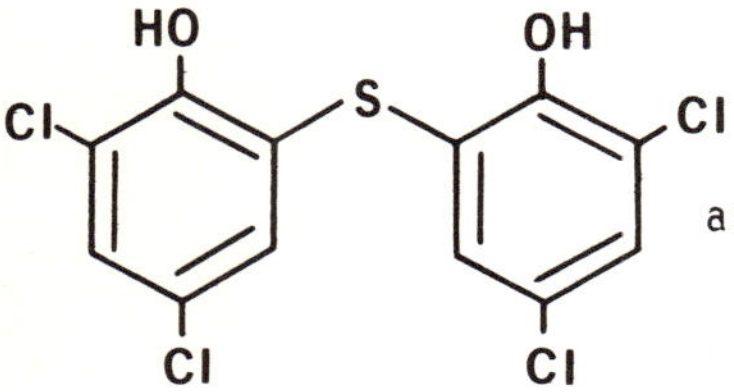

bithionol　　antiseptic　　chlorinated salicylanilide

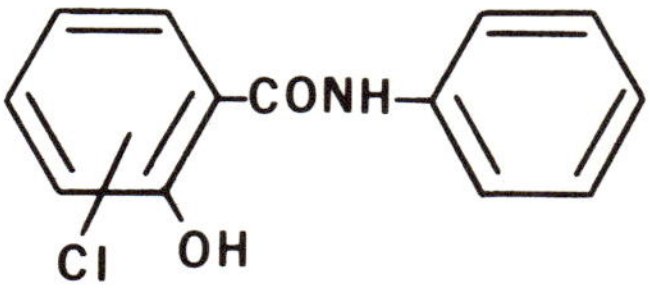

chloral hydrate　　ointments　　chlorobutanol

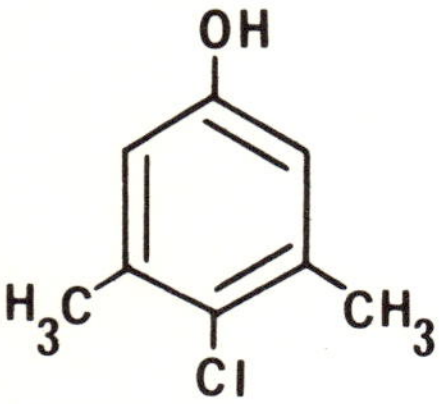

chloroxylenol　　creams, lotions　　chlorocresol

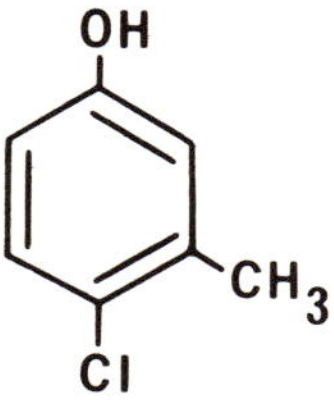

(continued)

Table 1 (continued)

Compound	Uses	Cross-reactant
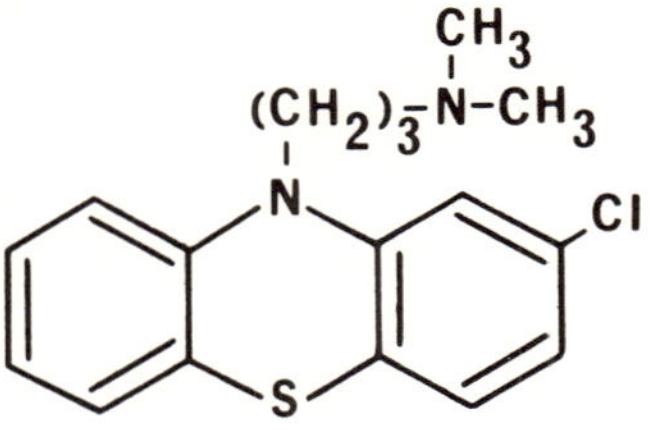 chlorpromazine	disinfectant	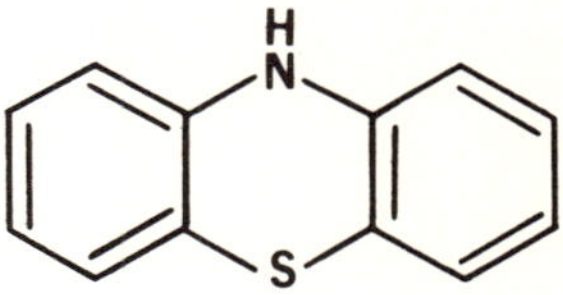 phenothiazine
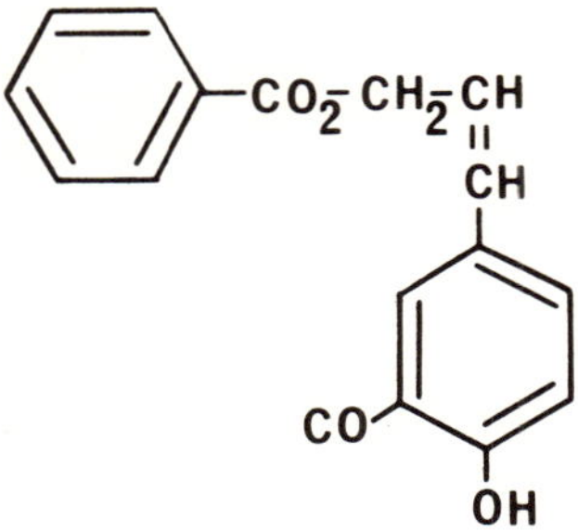 coniferyl benzoate	benzoin	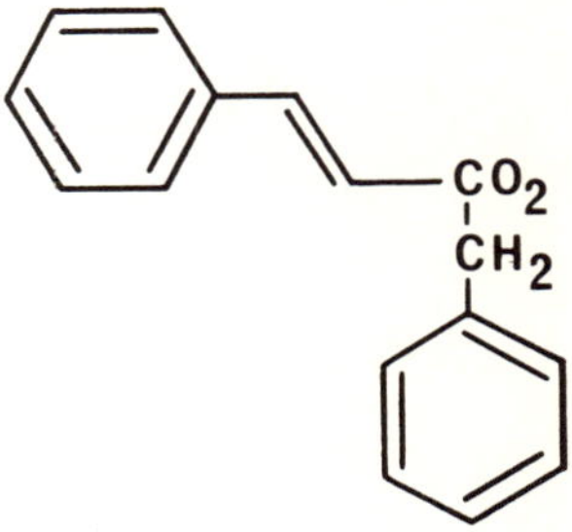 benzyl cinnamate
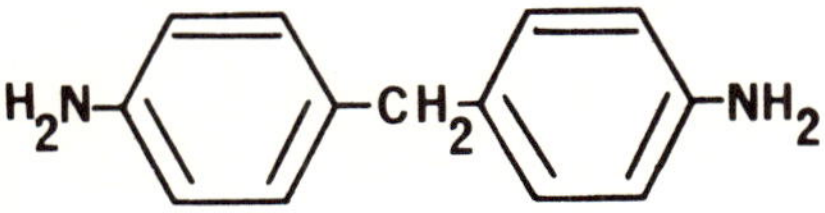 diaminodiphenylmethane	antioxidant	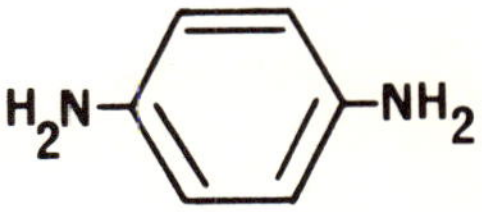 p-phenylenediamine (PPD)

(continued)

Table 1 (continued)

Compound	Uses	Cross-reactant

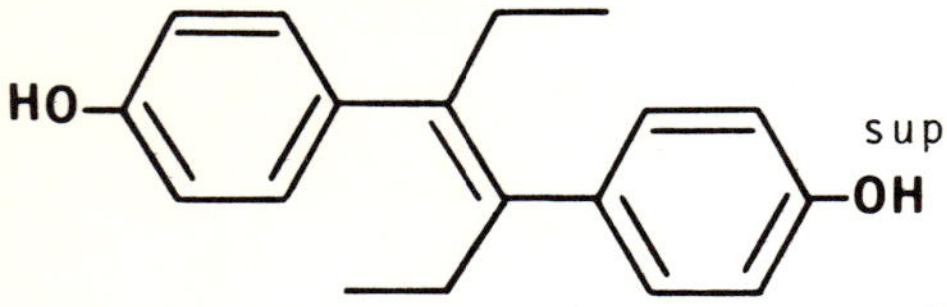

diethylstilbestrol

dienestrol

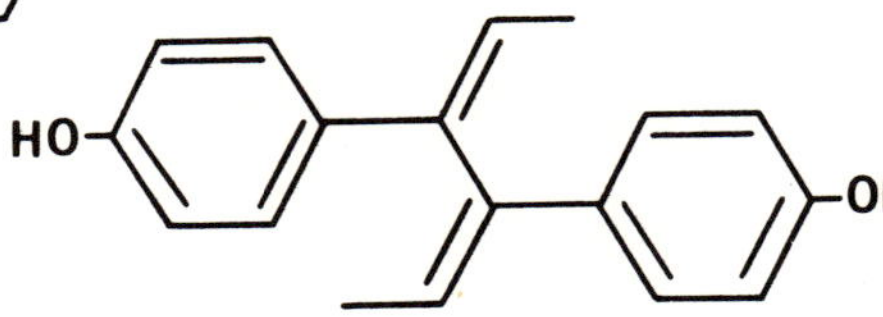

suppositories

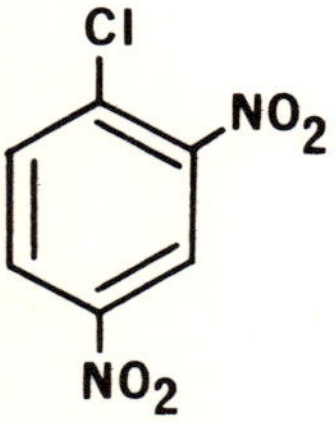

1-chloro-2,4-dinitrobenzene

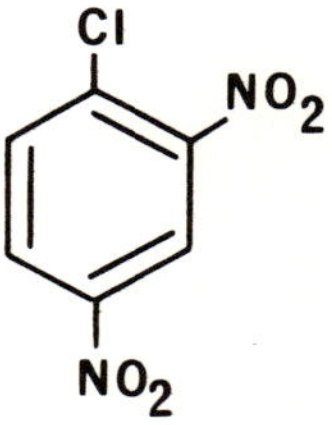

1-fluoro-2,4-dinitro-benzene

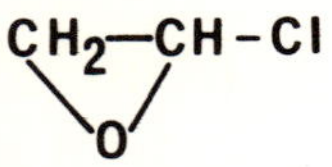

protein reagent, experimental contact allergy

epichlorhydrin

propylene oxide

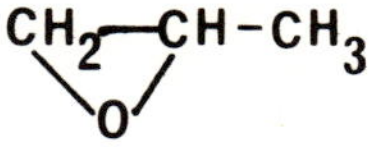

epoxy resins

ethylenediamine

antistine

creams, lotions

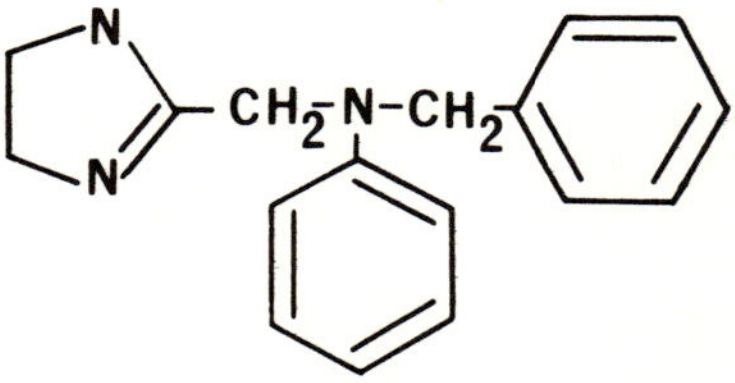

(continued)

Table 1 (continued)

Compound	Uses	Cross-reactant
fuschin (basic)	dye, antifungal agent	p-amino compounds
hexachlorophene	creams, oils, fungicide	bithionol
hexamethylenetetramine	antiseptic, rubber accelerator	HCHO formaldehyde
hexylresorcinol	creams, mouth wash	resorcinol

(continued)

Table 1 (continued)

Compound	Uses	Cross-reactant

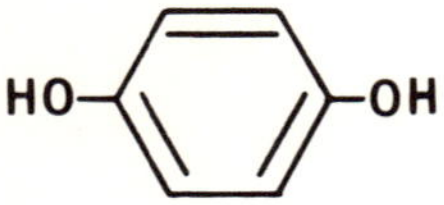

hydroquinone — antioxidant — pyrocatechol

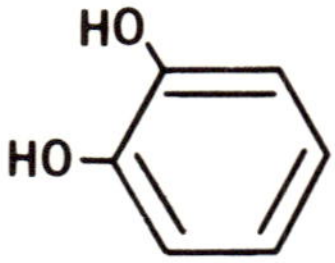

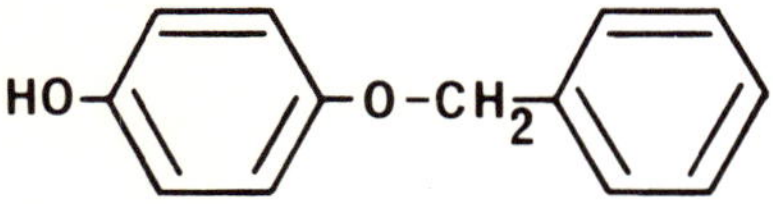

hydroquinone-O-benzyl ether (benoquin) — antioxidant, depigmenting agent — hydroquinone

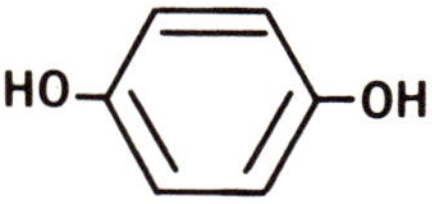

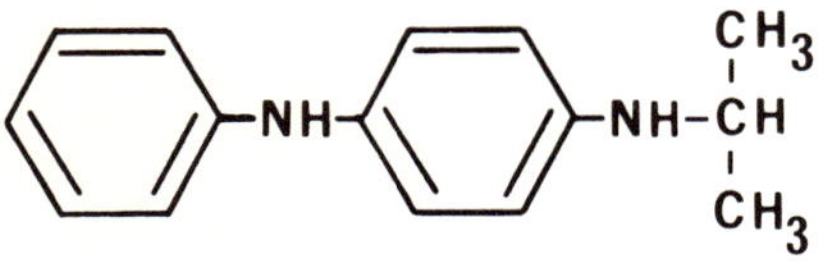

N-isopropyl-N'-phenyl-p-phenylenediamine — antioxidant — p-phenylenediamine

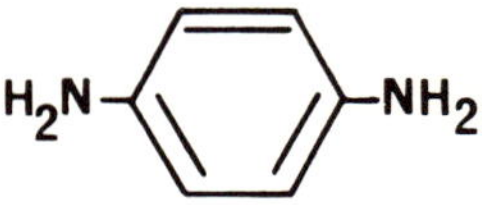

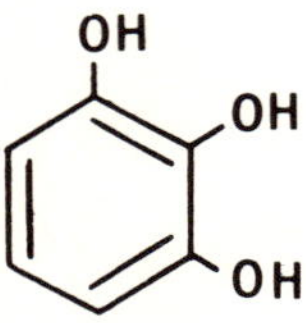

pyrogallol — dyes, tar — resorcinol

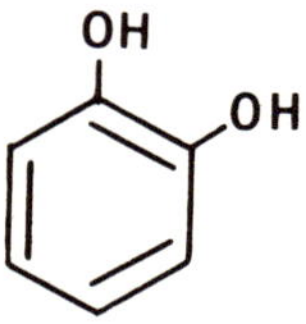

(continued)

Table 1 (continued)

Compound	Uses	Cross-reactant
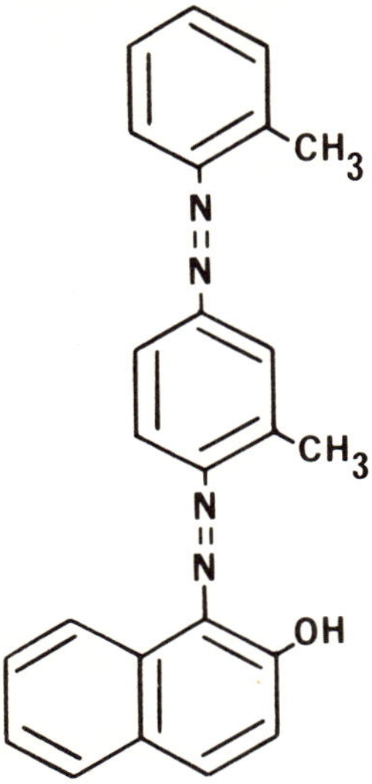 sudan IV	coloring agent	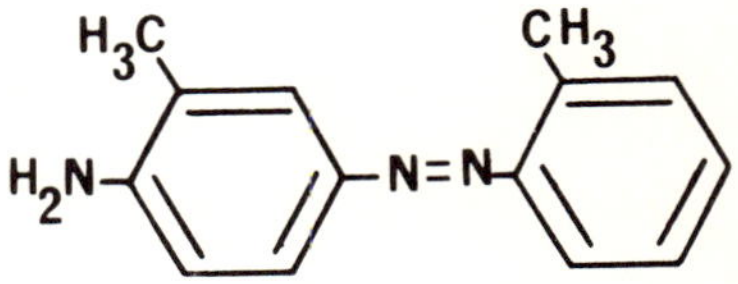 p-aminoazotoluene
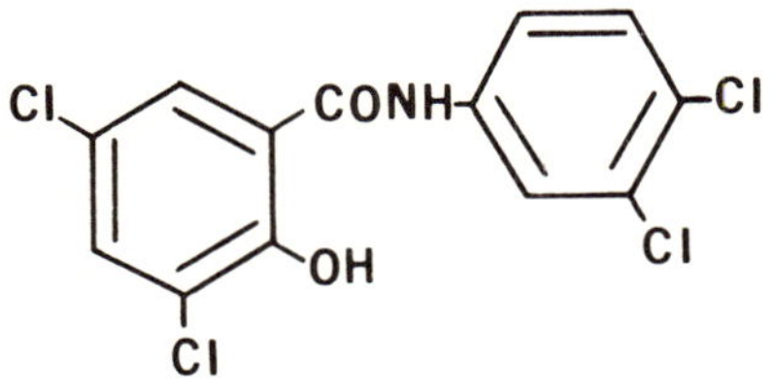 tetrachlorosalicylanilide (TCSA)	soaps	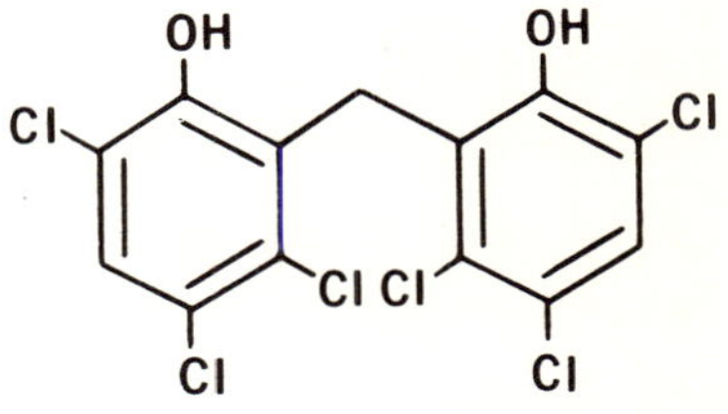 hexachlorophene
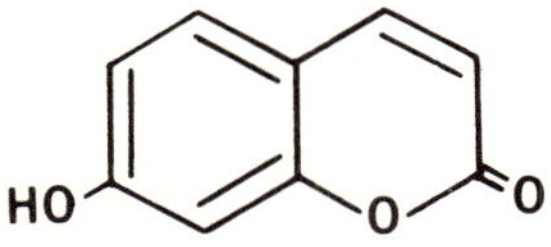 umbelliferone	sunscreening agent	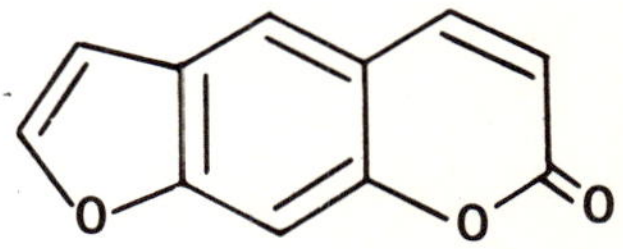 psoralen

(continued)

Table 1 (continued)

Compound	Uses	Cross-reactant

usnic acid — naturally occurring — atranorin

Table 2 Results of Patch-testing of Patients Sensitive to Diiodoquin or Vioform

	Patients		
Compounds	S	L	D
Quinoline (I)	–	–	–
Isoquinoline (II)	–	–	–
Quinaldine (III)	–	–	–
2-Chloroquinoline (IV)	–	–	–
8-Hydroxyquinoline (V)	4+	–	4+
Vioform (VI)	4+	4+	4+
Diiodoquin (VII)	4+	2+	2+
Quinolor (VIII)	4+	3+	4+
Sterosan (IX)	4+	1+	2+
Pyridine (X)	–	–	–
Nicotinic acid (XI)	2+	1+	4+
α-Picolinic acid (XII)	3+	2+	–
Quinolinic acid (XII)	3+	3+	4+

Patients were patch-tested with the compounds suspended in bland ointment (aquaphor) at varying concentrations.

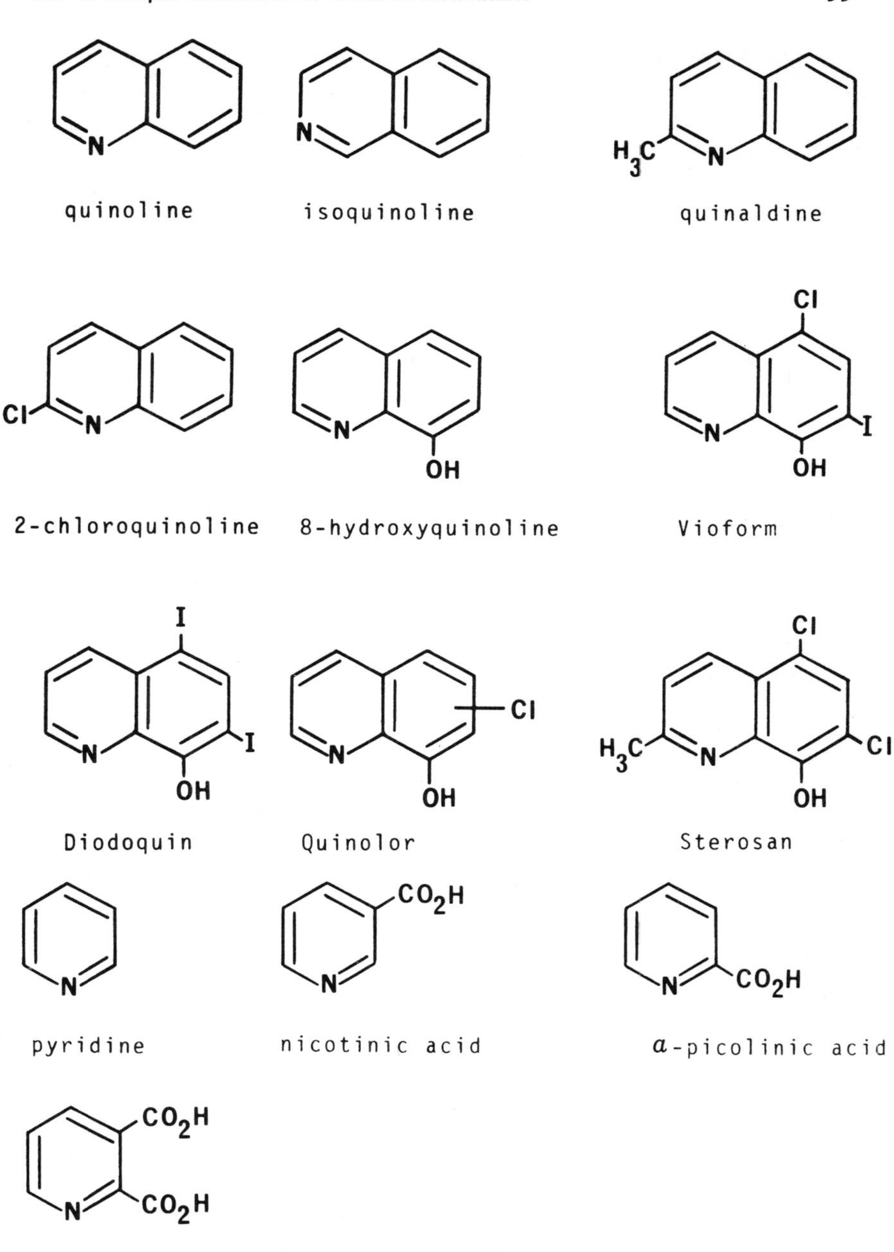

Figure 1 Chemical structures of the compounds listed in Table 2.

patch tests were conducted with carboxylated pyridines. Positive reactions
were observed for α-picolinic acid, nicotinic acid, and quinolinic acid. Pyridine itself did not give a positive result.

These results (patch-testing) strongly suggest that halogenated 8-hydroxy-
quinolines are unstable in these patients. In vivo chemical instability is not
surprising, in view of the fact that quinoline oxidation leads to preferential
oxidation of the benzene ring to yield the carboxylated pyridine (Hoogewerff
and van Dorp, 1879).

Hydroxylation in the 8 position will increase this susceptibility. It is also
interesting to note that α- or β-carboxy-substituted pyridines gave positive
reactions. Quinoline oxidation yields α- and β-carboxypyridines, and it is
possible that further in vivo degradation of this compound will give a mixture
of isomers (α and β), thus explaining cross-sensitization with α-picolonic and
nicotinic acids.

Oral administration of diiodoquin also resulted in a recrudescence of the
eczematous dermatitis after 12 hours.

Sesquiterpene Lactones

Sesquiterpene lactones have been identified as the main allergenic constituent
from plants belonging to the Compositae family (Mitchell et al., 1971; Mitchell
and Dupuis, 1971; Mitchell et al., 1972). These compounds vary widely in
terms of chemical functionalities, isomerism, basic carbon skeleton, and degree of oxidation (Yoshioka et al., 1973). Furthermore, some sesquiterpene
lactones can inhibit tumor growth (Hartwell and Abbott, 1969; Kupchan et
al., 1971; Lee et al., 1971; Rodriguez et al., 1976) and are cytotoxic (Dupuis
and Brisson, 1976; Schlewer et al., 1980b).

A structure-allergenicity study of these compounds has been reported
(Mitchell et al., 1970). In all compounds giving positive patch-test results in
sensitive patients, the presence of an α-methylene group conjugated to the
γ-lactone was necessary. The presence of the lactone ring was also important.
No general rules could be established, however, to explain cross-sensitization
or its absence. For instance, in patients sensitive to frullanolide, patients 1
and 2 gave a positive response to alantolactone, ludovicin A, B, and C,
eupatolide acetate, artemorin acetate, parthenolide, arbusculin A and B, and

Table 3 Cross-Reactivity between Sesquiterpene Lactones

	Patient	
Compound	1	2
Alantolactone (I)	3+	4+
Isoalantolactone (II)	–	±
Frullanolide (III)	2+	4+
Ludovicin A (IV)	4+	3+
Ludovicin B (V)	4+	4+
Ludovicin C (VI)	4+	4+
Eupatolide acetate (VII)	4+	2+
Artemorin acetate (VIII)	4+	2+
Parthenolide (IX)	4+	4+
Arbusculin A (X)	2+	3+
Arbusculin B (XI)	2+	1+
Coronopilin (XII)	2+	1+
Ambrosin (XIII)	3+	–
Cumambrin A (XIV)	3+	–
Cumambrin B (XV)	3+	–
Eupatoriopicrin (XVI)	4+	–
Chamissonin diacetate (XVII)	–	–
Xanthinin (XVIII)	–	–

Patients were patch-tested with solutions (30 μl) of the terpene in 80% aqueous alcohol. Reactions were read at 24 and 48 h and at 5 and 14 days.

Source: Data from Mitchell et al. (1970). © 1970 The Williams & Wilkins Co., Baltimore.

coronopilin. In addition, patient 1 reacted to ambrosin, cumambrin A and B, and eupatoriopicrin whereas patient 2 did not give a positive response. Negative responses were observed in both cases for compounds that possess "potential allergenicity," i.e., the properly substituted lactone ring. This was the case for isoalantolactone, xanthinin, and chamissonin diacetate (Table 3, Fig. 2).

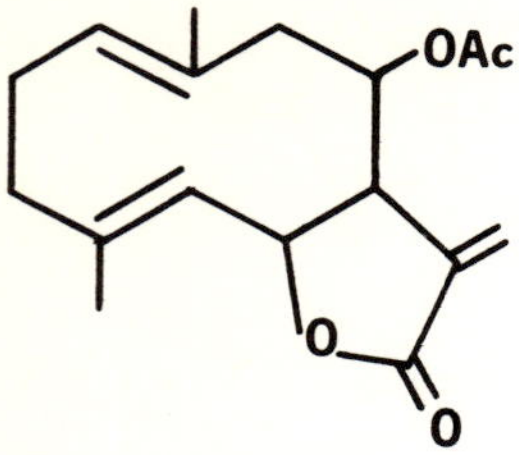

eupatolide acetate

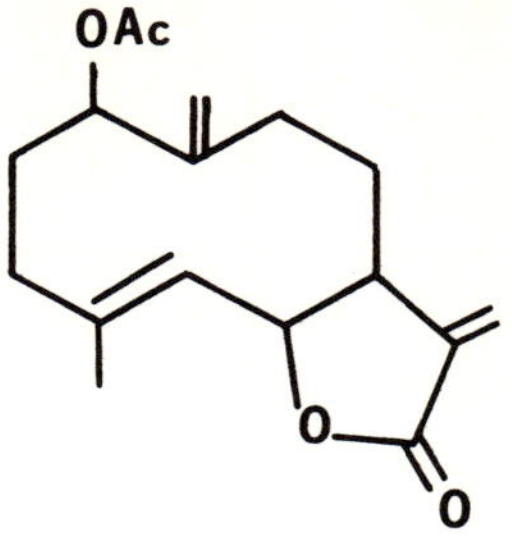

artemorin acetate

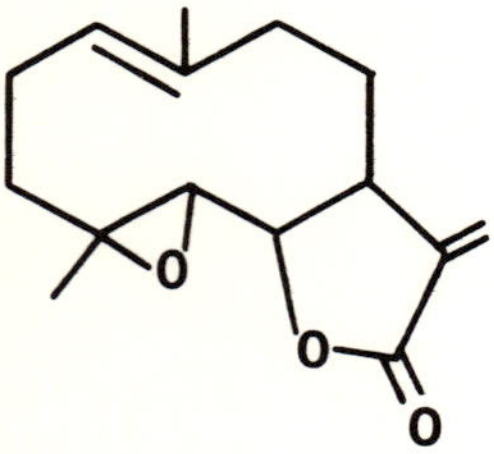

parthenolide

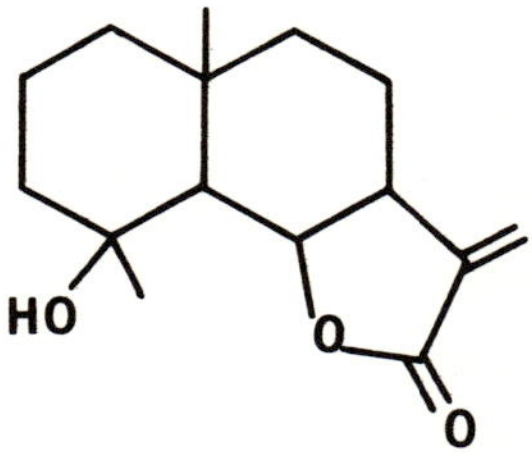

arbusculin-A

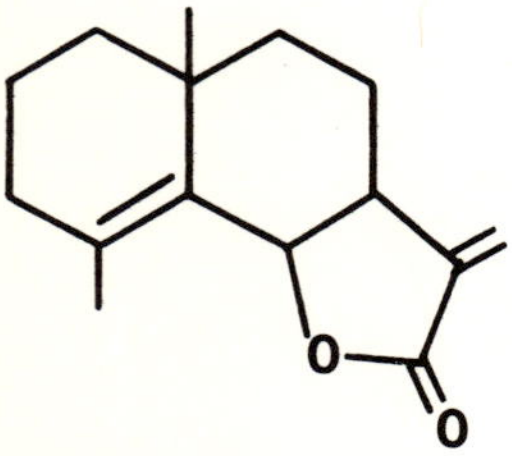

arbusculin-B

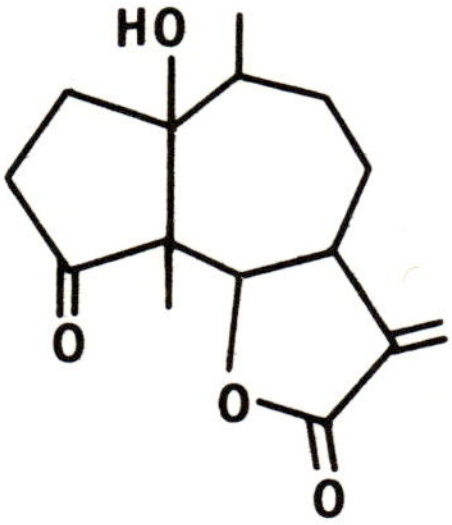

coronopilin

Figure 2 Chemical structures of the sesquiterpene lactones listed in Table 3.

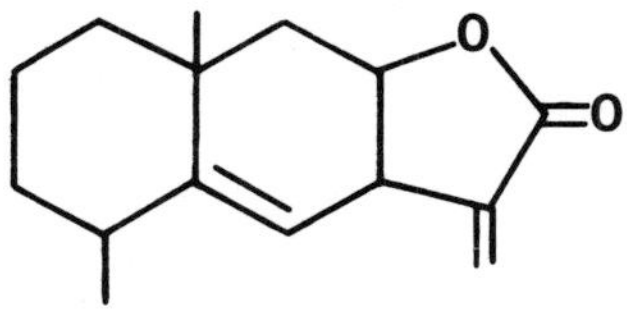

alantolactone

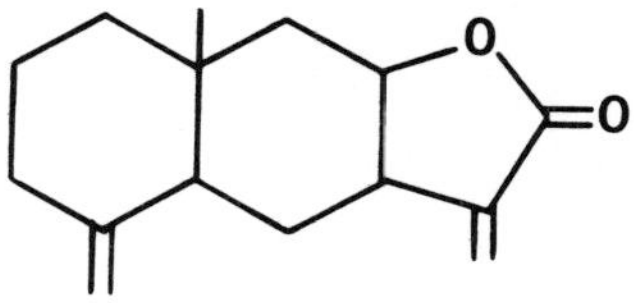

isoalantolactone

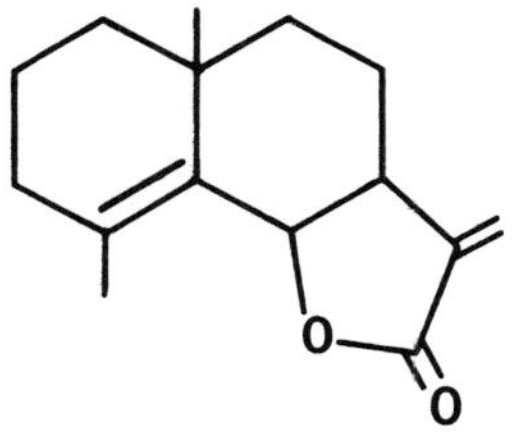

frullanolide

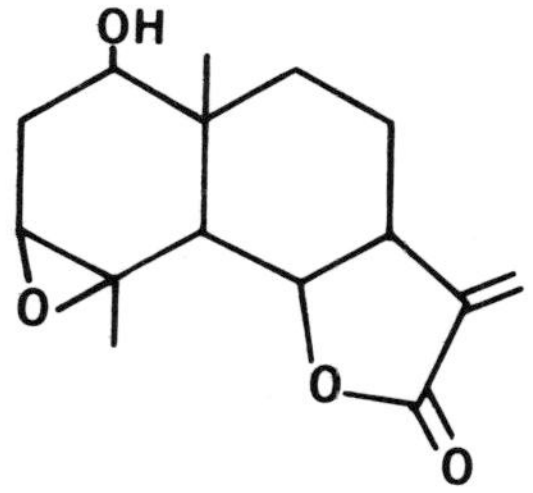

ludovicin-A

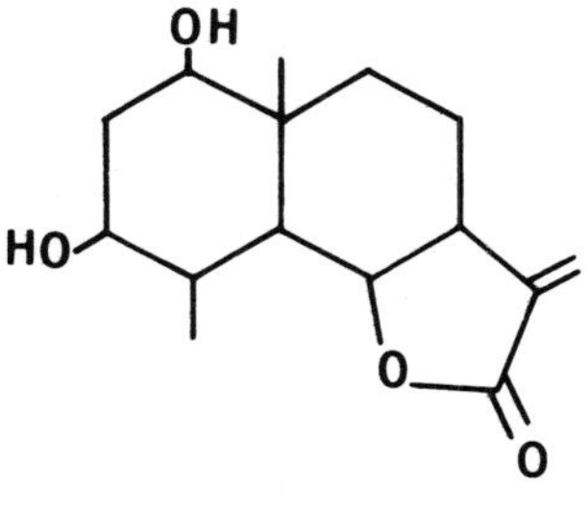

ludovicin-B

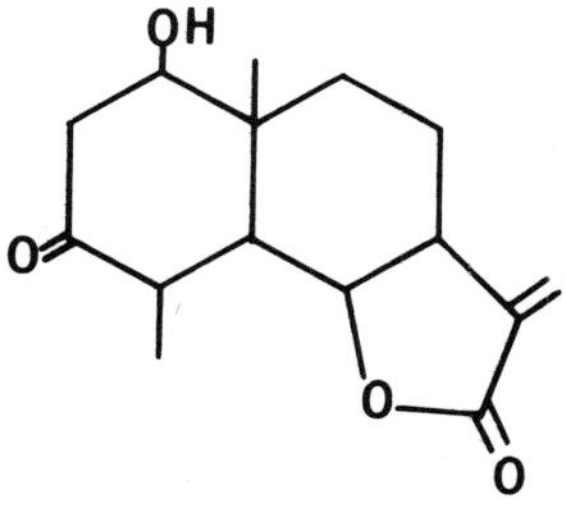

ludovicin-C

Figure 2 (continued)

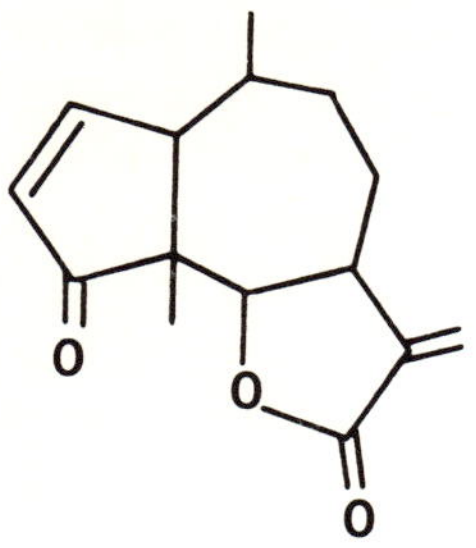

ambrosin

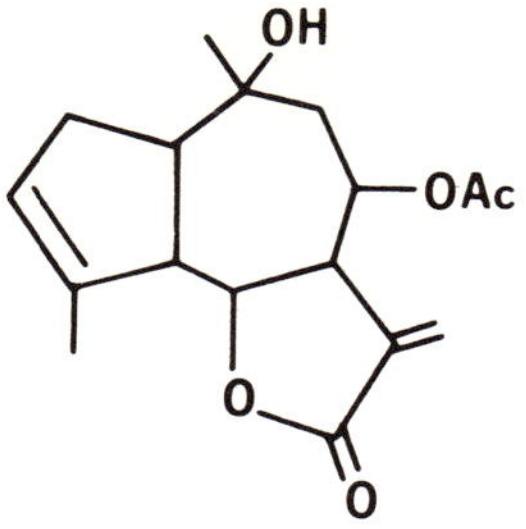

cumambrin-A

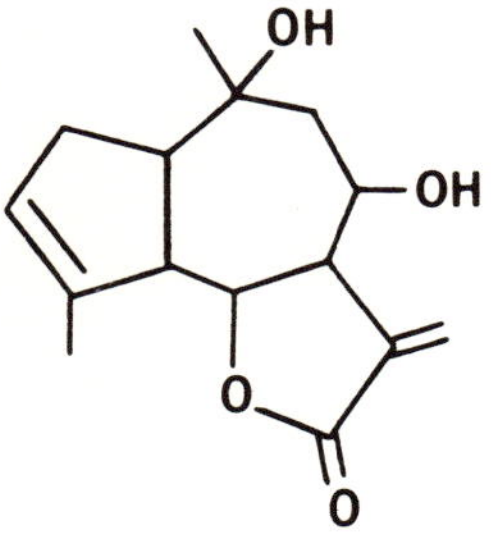

cumambrin-B

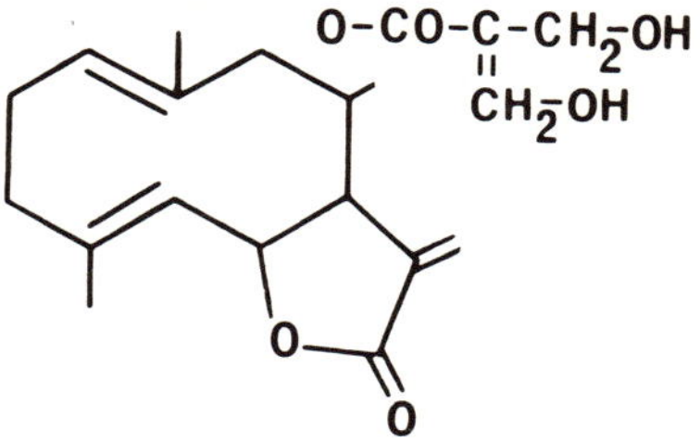

eupatoriopicrin

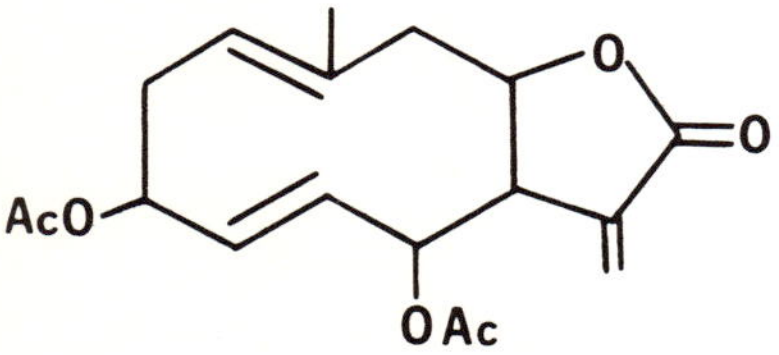

chamissonin diacetate

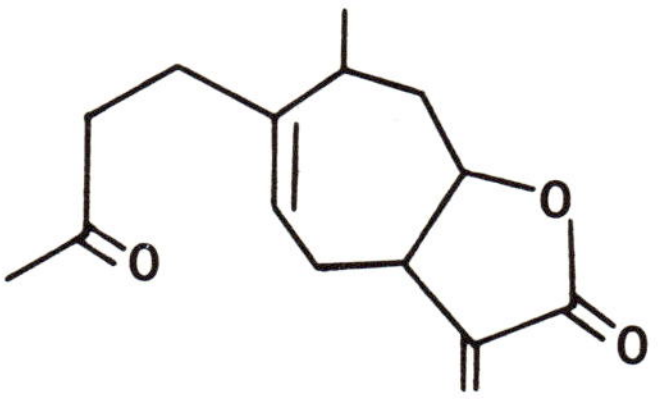

xanthinin

Figure 2 (continued)

It was concluded that cross-sensitization among sesquiterpene lactones depends not only on the nature of the hapten, but also on the "immunological specificity of the patient" tested (Mitchell et al., 1970). Compounds where the α-methylene group was reduced did not give positive patch tests in sensitive patients.

The metabolism of these compounds is unknown and it cannot be said if they are modified in vivo. The chemical interconversion of eudesmanolides to eremophilanolides has, however, been reported in vitro (Kitagawa et al., 1972, 1974).

Additional studies (Stampf et al., 1978) showed that there was also cross-reactivity between alantolactone and isoalantolactone in patients sensitive to *Frullania* (frullanolide) (Table 4, Fig. 3).

In a systematic study of ACD to α-methylene-γ-butyrolactones, Benezra's group showed (Schlewer et al., 1978; Stampf et al., 1978) that cross-reactivity exists between natural sesquiterpene lactones and synthetic lactones such as norbornene lactone, camphene spirolactone, and various γ, γ-disubstituted α-methylene-γ-butyrolactones (see Table 6). It was also demonstrated that patients allergic to frullanolide or that guinea pigs sensitized to alantolactone did not react to α-methylene-γ-butyrolactone. This observation would suggest that, along with subtle structure-activity relationships, solubility could play an important role in determining the sensitizing capacity of lactones: a lipophilic part seems essential for activity. α-Methylene-γ-butyrolactone is a water-soluble compound, whereas sesquiterpenes are liposoluble compounds. It is possible, however, to sensitize guinea pigs to α-methylene-γ-butyrolactone itself (Schlewer et al., 1980a).

Para-Nitro Compounds

Cross-sensitization to *para*-nitro compounds, such as *p*-nitrophenol or Mintacol, has been reported (Foussereau and Benezra, 1970, 1982). This cross-sensitization appears to be rare and much less frequent than cross-sensitivity to *para*-amino compounds. *Para*-nitro compounds and *para*-amino compounds may give by in vivo transformation similar intermediates, which could be transformed into quinones.

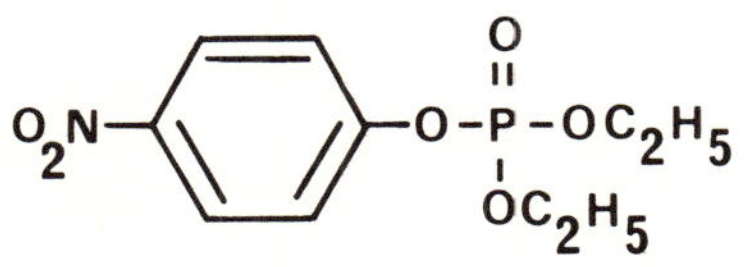

Mintacol

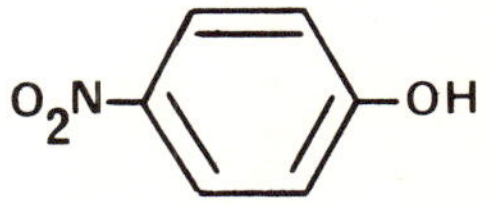

p-nitrophenol

Table 4 Cross-Reactivity between Sesquiterpene Lactones in Patients Sensitive to *Frullania*

| | Intensities of skin reaction | | | | | | |
| | Patients | | | | | | |
Compounds tested	1	2	3	4	5	6	Average
Alantolactone (I)	1+	0	1+	3+	1+	±	1.0
Isoalantolactone (II)	0	0	0	3+	1+	1+	0.8
α-Methylene-γ-butyrolactone (III)	N.T.[a]	0	0	0	0	N.T.	0
Norbornane lactone (IV)	1+	0	0	0	1+	1+	0.5
Spirolactone (V)	1+	1+	1+	1+	1+	1+	1.0
Frullanolide (VI)	1+	1+	3+	3+	1+	1+	1.6
Frullania	N.T.	2+	2+	3+	2+	N.T.	2.2

[a]N.T., not tested.

Patch-testing was done with the lactones in alcoholic (0.1%) solution. Results were read at 48 hr.

Source: From Stampf et al. (1978).

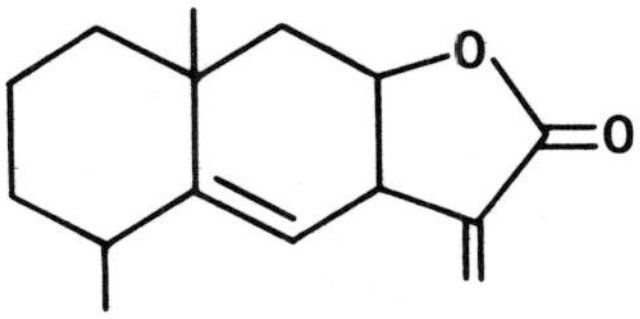

alantolactone

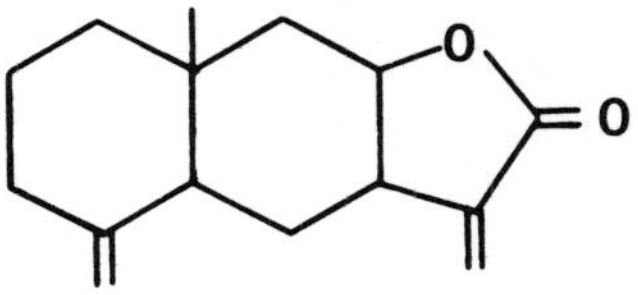

isoalantolactone

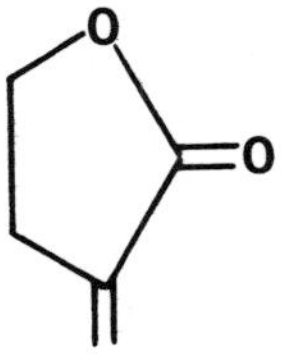

α-methylene-γ-butyrolactone

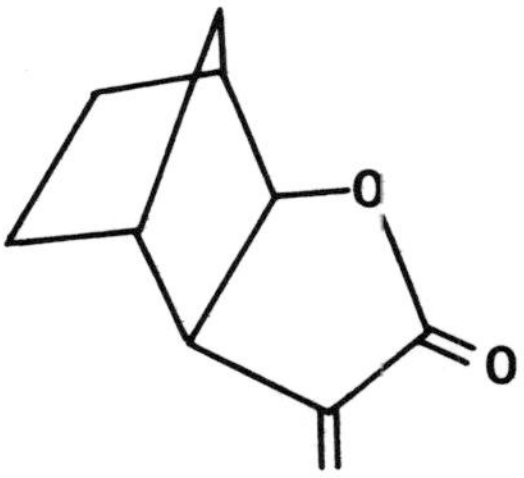

norbornane lactone

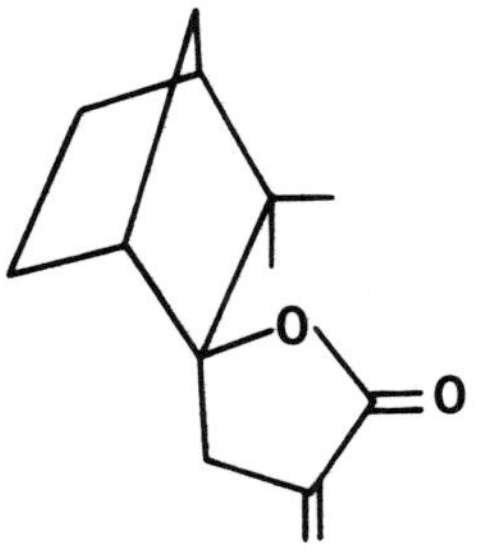

camphene spirolactone

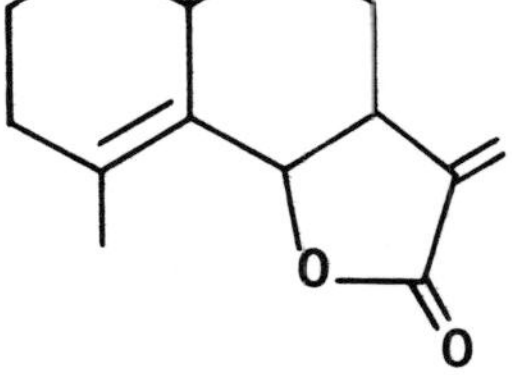

frullanolide

Figure 3 Chemical structures of the lactones listed in Table 4.

Phenolic Compounds

Cross-sensitivity between diethylstilbestrol (DES) and other biphenols has
been reported (Fregert and Rorsman, 1960). The study was performed with
one patient sensitive to DES. Cross-reactivity with a series of phenolic compounds was investigated and is illustrated by some examples in Table 5.

Examination of the chemical structures (Fig. 4) does not reveal obvious
reasons to explain reactivity towards certain compounds and absence of reaction to others. For instance, the patient reacted to DES but failed to give
a positive patch test to stilbene. It can be argued that the presence of ethyl
groups is necessary. This does not appear to be the case, however, since *p*-
benzylphenol gives a positive skin reaction. The reason for this observation
may be that stilbene is a poor substrate for *p*-hydroxylation. Positive reaction
to eugenol would tend to suggest that the DES molecule is cleaved to give a
phenol derivative. Failure to give this derivative would explain negative reactions to dihydroxydiphenyl and benzestrol.

Table 5 Cross-Reactivity between Diethylstilbestrol and Other Compounds

Compound	Patch-test results
Dienestrol (II)	positive
Hexestrol (III)	positive
Bisphenol A (IV)	positive
Diethylstilbestrol monomethyl ether (V)	positive
p-Benzylphenol (VI)	positive
Hydroquinone monobenzyl ether (VII)	positive
Eugenol (VIII)	positive
Dihydroxydiphenyl (IX)	negative
Benzestrol (X)	negative
Stilbene (XI)	negative
Benzophenone (XII)	negative
Phloretin (XIII)	negative
Rosalic acid (XIV)	negative

The patient developed sensitivity to a hair lotion containing diethylstilbestrol. Cross-
reactivity was tested to the compounds listed above dissolved in ethanol.
Source: Data from Fregert and Rorsman (1960).

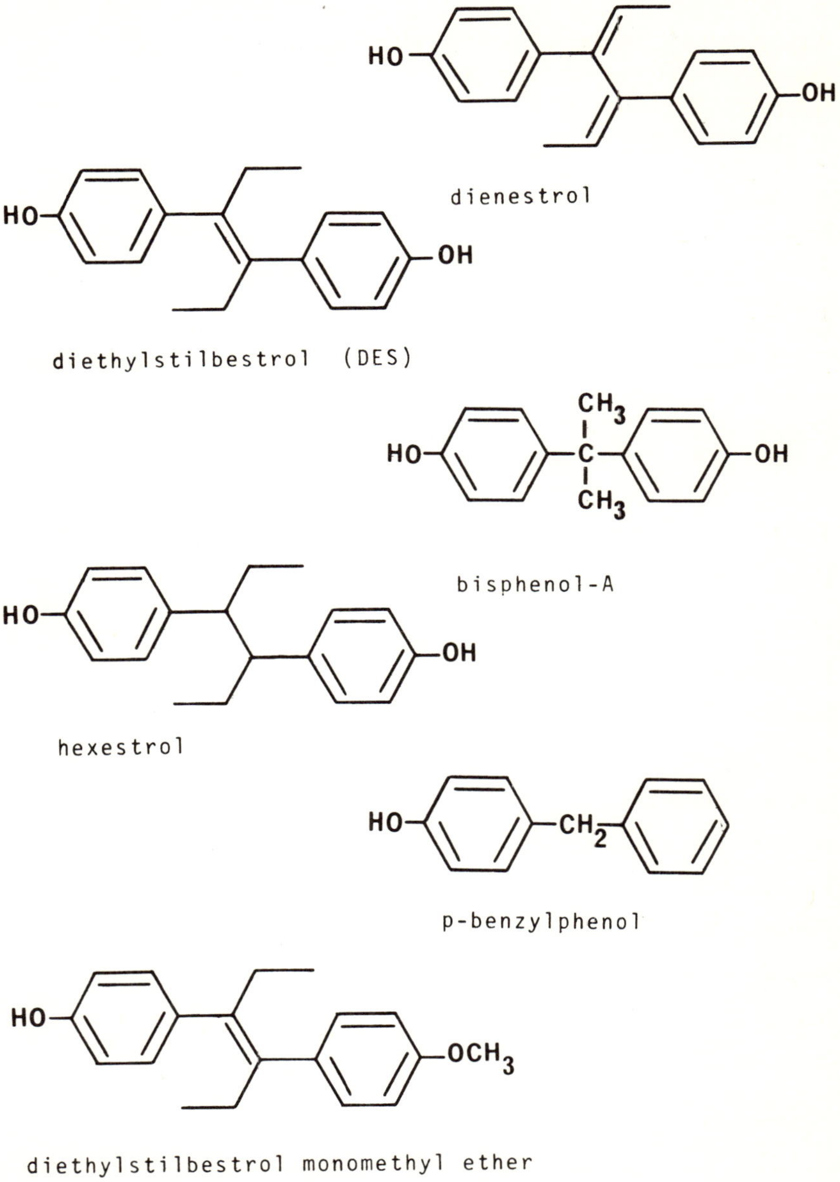

Figure 4 Chemical structures of the compounds listed in Table 5.

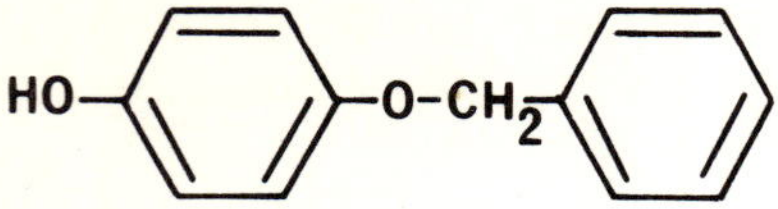

hydroquinone monobenzyl ether 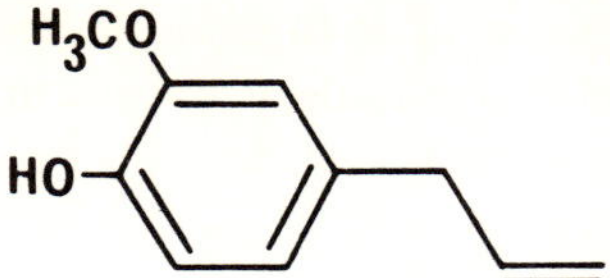   eugenol

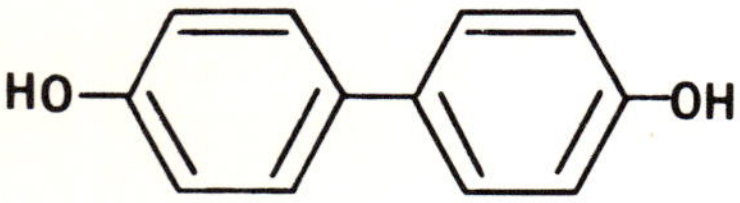

dihydroxydiphenyl 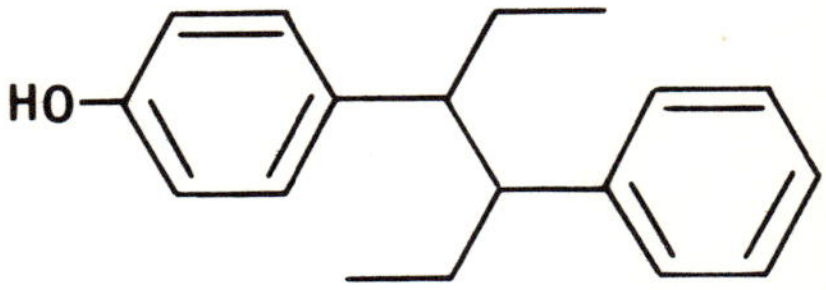   benzestrol

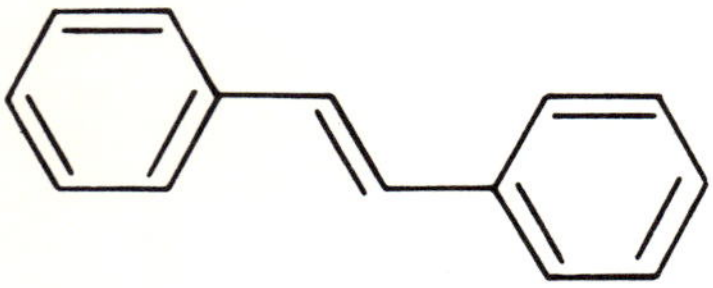

stilbene 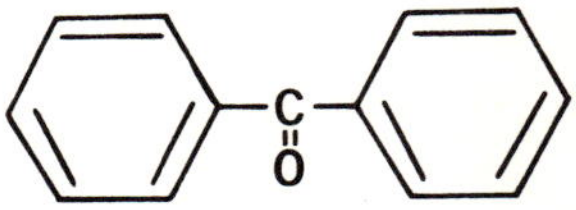   benzophenone

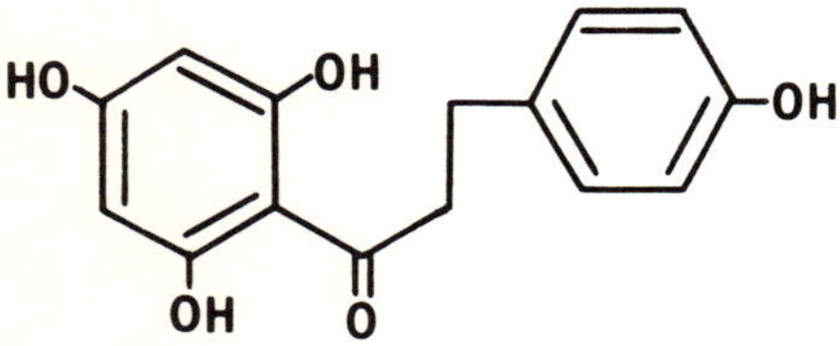

phloretin 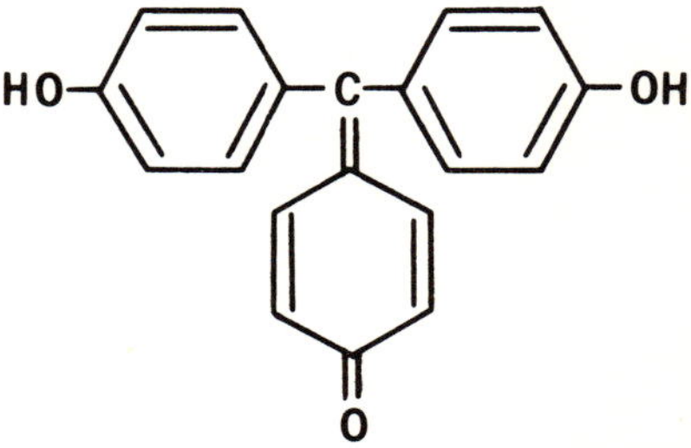   rosalic acid

Figure 4 (continued)

The case of phloretin is interesting. This phenolic compound can be degraded into phloroglucinol and dihydrocoumaric acid. This degradation has been reported, however, only by some fungal systems (Minamikawa et al., 1970).

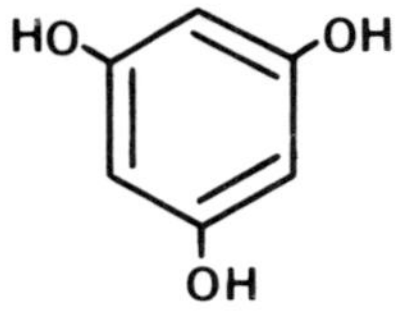

phloroglucinol 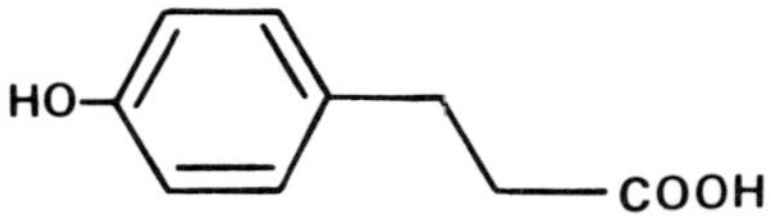   dihydrocoumaric acid

Para-amino Compounds

Substituted Anilines

Cross-sensitization between 1,4-disubstituted aromatic amines has been reported (Nitti et al., 1937). In addition, cross-reaction between *para*-amino compounds and aniline or *p*-phenylenediamine (PPD), may result, as suggested by Mayer (1930, 1950), from formation of a common oxidation product.

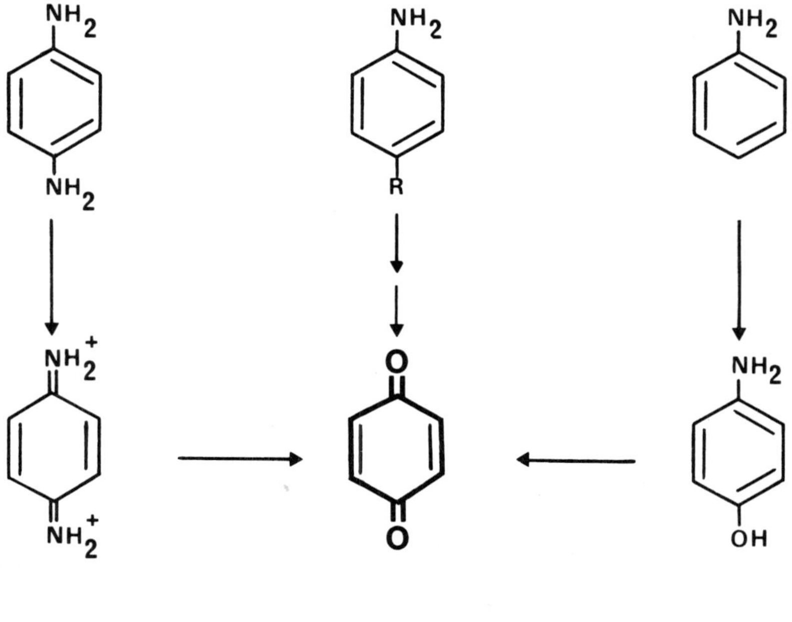

Compounds of the type $NH_2\text{-}C_6H_4\text{-}R$, where R is CO_2H, $CO_2C_2H_5$, glycerol, or SO_2NH_2, have been extensively studied (Meltzer and Baer, 1949; Schulz, 1960). In one patient strongly sensitive to benzocaine, strong positive responses were observed for butesin ($R = CO_2C_4H_9$), p-aminobenzoic acid ($R = CO_2H$), PPD ($R = NH_2$), aniline ($R = H$), and procaine [$R = CO_2C_2H_4N(C_2H_5)_2$]. Compounds lacking a *para*-amino function were negative. *P*-Nitrobenzoic acid gave a negative patch-test result.

Sulfonamides

A study of substituted sulfonamides (Schulz, 1960) showed that when the amino function was separated from the aromatic nucleus by a spacer, the frequency of positive response decreased.

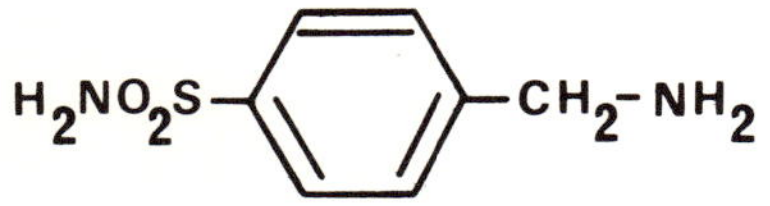

$$H_2NO_2S\text{---}\langle C_6H_4 \rangle\text{---}CH_2\text{-}NH_2$$

aminomethylsulfonamide   (7 positive cases)

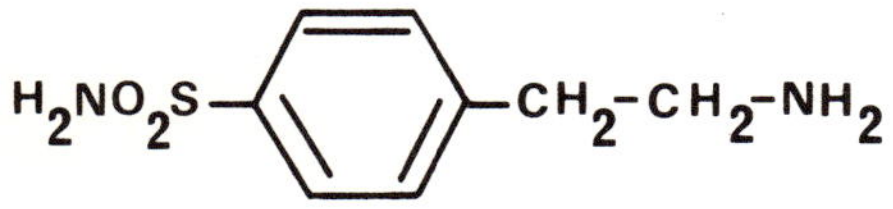

$$H_2NO_2S\text{---}\langle C_6H_4 \rangle\text{---}CH_2\text{-}CH_2\text{-}NH_2$$

aminoethylsulfonamide   (5 positive cases)

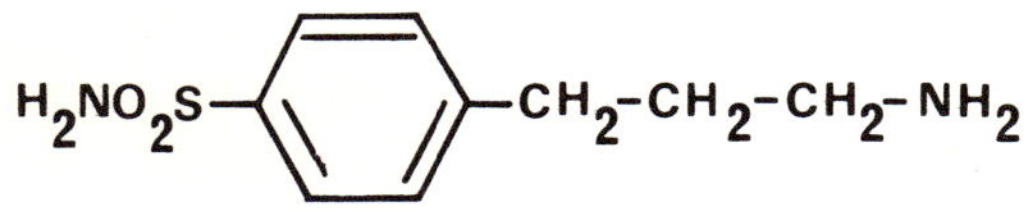

$$H_2NO_2S\text{---}\langle C_6H_4 \rangle\text{---}CH_2\text{-}CH_2\text{-}CH_2\text{-}NH_2$$

aminopropylsulfonamide   (2 positive cases)

Azo Dyes

Artificial coloring agents, such as azo dyes, are widely used in food, cosmetics, and in the textile industry. Allergic reactions to these compounds are fairly common (Zina and Bonu, 1965), as well as cross-reactions between them. Most important, is the frequent observation that patients sensitive to azo dyes also give a positive reaction to PPD. Cross-reaction between PPD and azo dyes has been observed for methyl red, aminoazotoluene, and its acetyl derivatives (Zina and Bonu, 1965). These observations lent support to Mayer's quinone theory (Mayer, 1950).

methyl red   aminoazotoluene

In a study of seven patients strongly sensitive to PPD, Baer (1954) reported cross-sensitization to aniline, FD & C Yellow 6, acetamine yellow, acetamine scarlet, and p-aminobenzoic acid and a weak or negative reaction to anthranilic acid, m-aminobenzoic acid, 3,5-dinitrobenzoic acid, procaine, and sulfanil-amide. In patients showing a weak reaction to PPD, only benzocaine gave consistently weak positive responses.

FD & C Yellow 6

Examination of the chemical structures of these allergens reveals that (if one assumes in vivo degradation of the dye yellow 6 to p-amino sulfonic acid and o-amino naphthol) further oxidation of the sulfonic acid to p-quinone explains the patient's cross-reaction to PPD (7 positive cases), aniline (5 positive cases), o- and p-aminobenzoic acid (5 positive and 4 positive cases, respectively), benzocaine (3 positive cases), and procaine (3 positive cases). Failure of pantocaine to give a positive patch test could be due to the N-alkyl substitution of the molecule which, in these patients, is not easily oxidized.

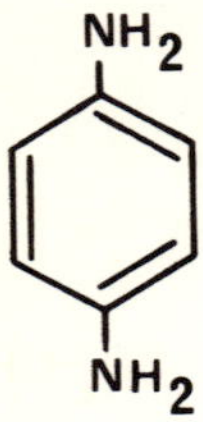

PPD   (7 positive cases)

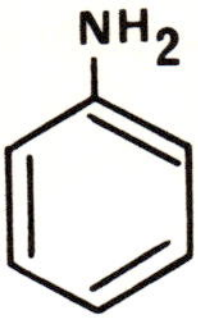

aniline
(5 positive cases)

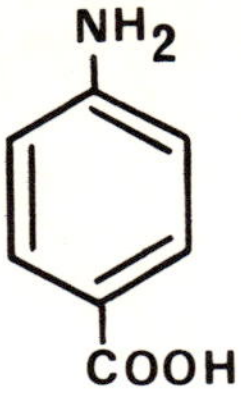

p-aminobenzoic acid
(5 positive cases)

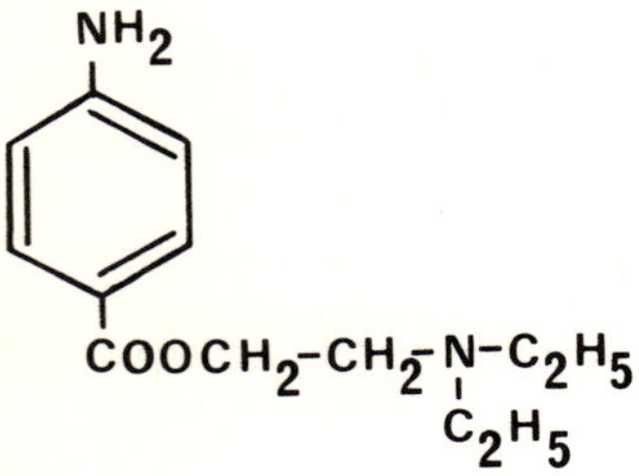

procaine   (3 positive cases)

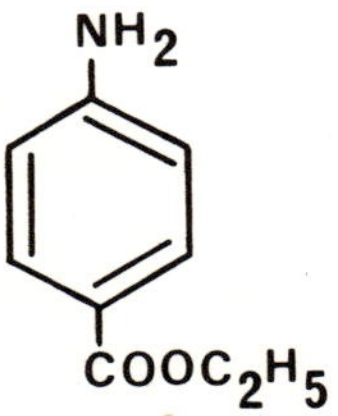

benzocaine   (3 positive cases)

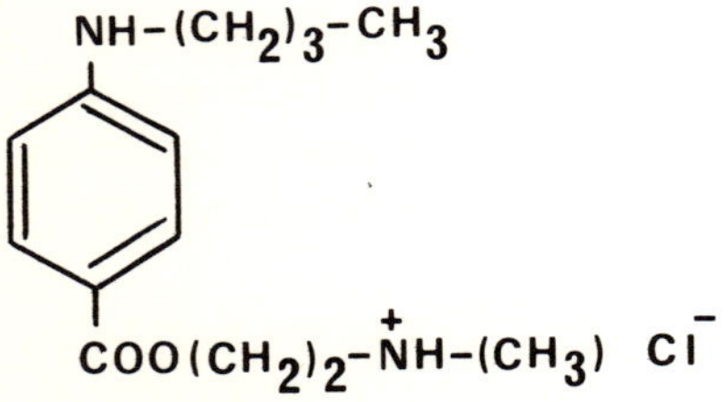

prontocaine

Local Anesthetics

Cross-sensitization to local anesthetics of the procaine type is difficult to rationalize. These compounds can undergo several in vivo chemical degradations, as illustrated:

$$H_2N-\langle\rangle-COO(CH_2)_2-N(C_2H_5)_2$$

procaine

$$H_2N-\langle\rangle-COO-CH_2-CHO$$

$$H_2N-\langle\rangle-COOH \quad + \quad HO-CH_2-CH_2-\underset{(C_2H_5)_2}{N}$$

p-aminobenzoic acid

$$OHC-CHO$$

glyoxal

$$O=\langle\rangle=O \quad \longleftarrow \quad HO-\langle\rangle-COOH$$

benzoquinone   p-hydroxybenzoic acid

It is not surprising, therefore, that patients sensitive to procaine have been reported to be also sensitive to *p*-hydroxybenzoic acid (Schwarzschild, 1928), to *N,N*-diethylaminoethane (James, 1931), to dialkylbenzoate esters (Waldron, 1934), to *p*-aminobenzoic acid (Goodman, 1941), and to alkyl esters of *p*-aminobenzoic acid.

The results of these studies emphasize the importance of the knowledge of the possible in vivo pathways of hapten modifications for a carefully planned study of cross-sensitization to low-molecular-weight chemicals.

Catechol Derivatives

Cross-sensitization to catechols seems to be related to ease of oxidation of these compounds into quinones. For instance, hydroquinone is a stronger sensitizer than pyrocatechol or resorcinol. Cross-reactivity among these compounds has been reported to be more frequent in the case of hydroquinone pyrocatechol than in the case of hydroquinone resorcinol (Sidi et al., 1964).

hydroquinone   pyrocatechol   resorcinol

If catechol oxidation is prevented by methoxylation, sensitization and cross-reaction may be prevented. Benzylation, which yields a less chemically stable group, is not effective against immunological reactivity to catechols.

The catechol derivatives from poison ivy are one of the most potent of the naturally occurring allergens (Dawson, 1956; Johnson et al., 1972; Kligman, 1958; Markiewitz and Dawson, 1965; Symes and Dawson, 1954). A structure-allergenicity relationship of various alkylated (on the benzene ring) catechols (Fig. 5) has been reported in humans (Keil et al., 1944; Kligman, 1958) and in quinea pigs (Baer et al., 1966, 1968, 1970). Table 6 illustrates the studies done in humans.

Table 6 Structure-Allergenicity Relationships of Catechol Derivatives

Compound	Number of positive responses/number of patients tested	Average intensity of positive reactions
Rhus leaves	19/21	+2
3-Pentadecylcatechol	21/21	+3
4-Pentadecylcatechol	8/21	+1
Urushiol dimethylether	3/13	+2/+3
3-Pentadecenyl-1′-veratrole	3/14	+2
3-Methylcatechol	3/21	+1/+2
3-Geranylcatechol	2/2	+4

Individuals were initially tested to poison ivy *Rhus* leaves or an extract of the plant or both. Twenty one persons showed a positive patch-test reaction and they were selected for the study.
Source: From Keil et al. (1944).

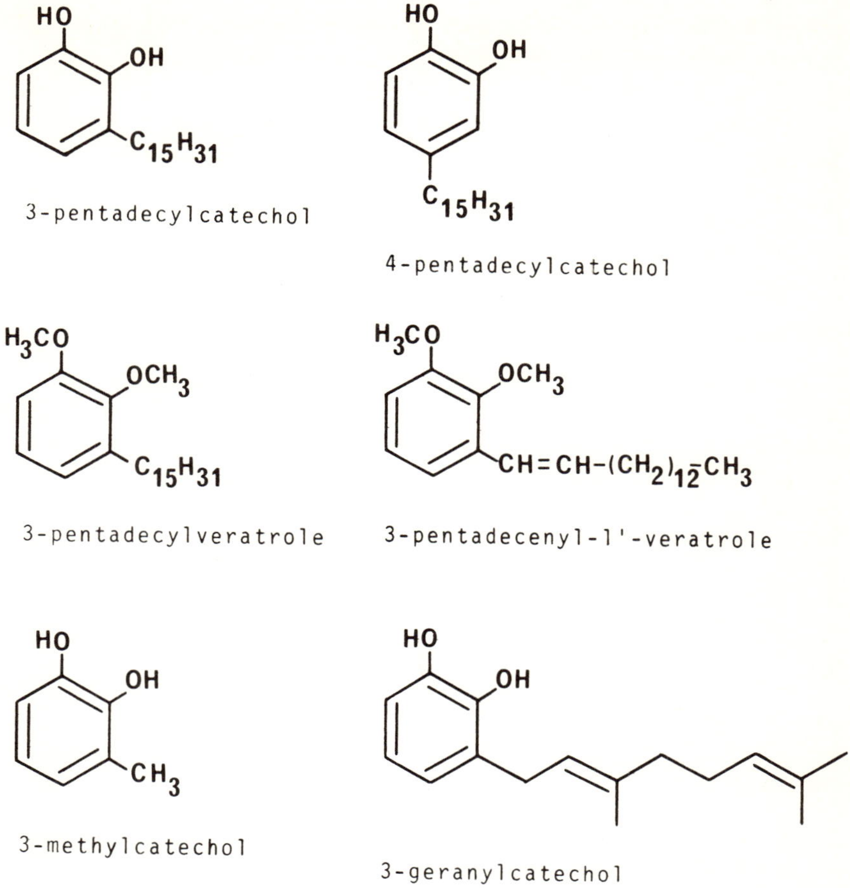
HO
OH
$C_{15}H_{31}$
3-pentadecylcatechol
HO
OH
$C_{15}H_{31}$
4-pentadecylcatechol
H_3CO
OCH_3
$C_{15}H_{31}$
3-pentadecylveratrole
H_3CO
OCH_3
$CH=CH-(CH_2)_{12}-CH_3$
3-pentadecenyl-1'-veratrole
HO
OH
CH_3
3-methylcatechol
HO
OH
3-geranylcatechol

Figure 5 Chemical structures of the catechol derivatives listed in Table 6.

These results indicate that a cross-reaction between urushiol and the substituted catechols depends on a minimum alkyl chain length and on the hydrophobicity of the side chain. The position of the alkyl side chain also influences cross-reaction.

Piperazine Derivatives

Cross-sensitization to piperazine and piperazine derivatives is related to the presence of two unsubstituted nitrogen atoms in the six-membered ring (Foussereau, 1963; Foussereau and Benezra, 1967). For instance, in patients sensitive to piperazine, the frequency of reaction decreases when the nitrogens are methylated as illustrated below.

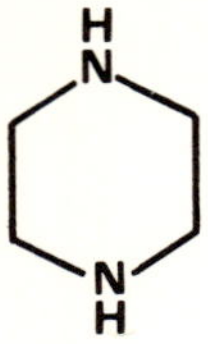

piperazine
(6 positive cases)

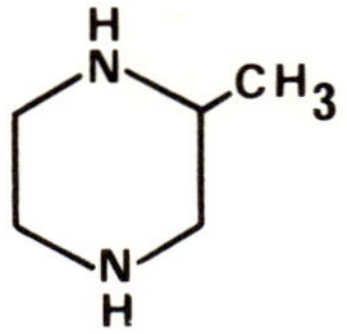

2-methylpiperazine
(5 positive cases)

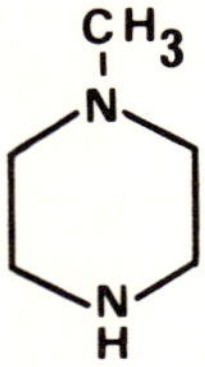

N-methylpiperazine
(3 positive cases)

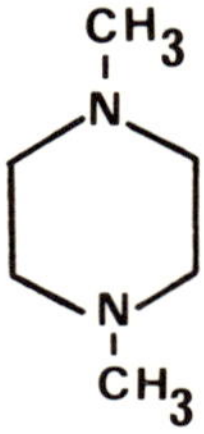

N,N'-dimethylpiperazine
(1 positive case)

These observations are probably related to decreasing ease of oxidation of the *N*-substituted piperazines.

Antioxidants

Antioxidants are added to foods, cosmetics, and pharmaceuticals to prevent oxidation of unsaturated fatty acids, which yields products with unpleasant flavor and rancid taste.

In the case of six patients sensitive to nordihydroguaiaretic acid (NDGA), Roed-Petersen and Hjorth (1976) have reported a cross-reaction to butylated hydroxyanisole (BHA) and/or butylated hydroxytoluene (BHT).

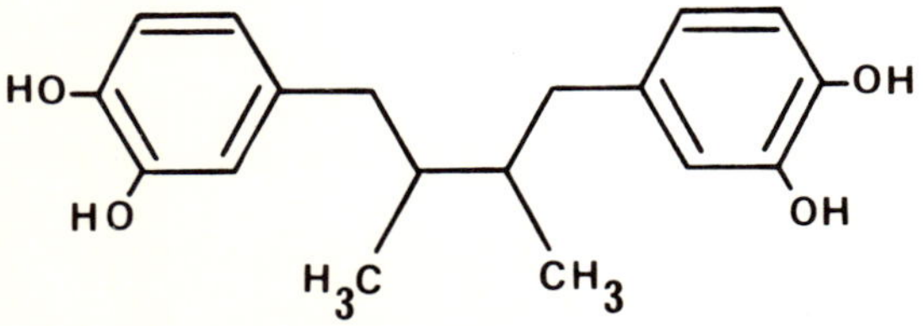

NDGA

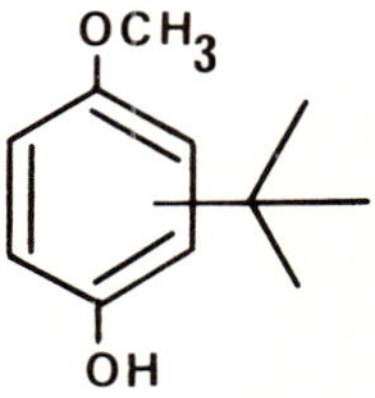

BHA

Cross-reaction between NDGA and BHA is explainable on the basis of the former giving an *o*-quinone structure and the latter a *p*-quinone. The presence of a diquinone structure does not seem to be essential (NDGA) and this may suggest a cleavage of NDGA into two molecules of 4-propyl catechol. Positive reactions to BHT are not easily explained. One has to assume that proper oxidation of BHT yields a *p*-quinone. This oxidation is certainly hampered by the presence of two bulky tertiary butyl groups on the benzene ring.

Usnic acid

The Role of Configuration

A study of seven patients sensitive to usnic acid revealed that only *d*-usnic acid gave positive patch tests (Mitchell, 1965, 1966; Mitchell and Shibata, 1969). These studies have been confirmed in guinea pigs (Hausen, personal communication). The *l*-isomer was, in each study, inactive. Interestingly, when the double bond in position 4,4a was reduced, *l*-dihydrousnic acid gave positive patch tests. *d*-Dihydrousnic acid was not tested.

dihydrousnic acid

Usnic acid is an optically active molecule because of the presence of a chiral (asymmetric) carbon atom at position 9b. The molecule possesses several electrophilic systems where nucleophilic addition ($\rightarrow$) can occur.

Nucleophilic addition at position 4a can be eliminated right away as a site of attachment to proteins because dihydro-4,4a-usnic acid shows positive patch tests, suggesting that the double bond (4,4a) conjugated to the carbonyl is not essential.

Reaction of usnic acid with amines occurs at positions 11 and 13 of the acetyl groups (Kutney and Sanchez, 1976). If a similar reaction occurs in vivo, the ensuing *d*-usnic acid-protein adduct could be specifically recognized by the immune system. The ability of the immune system to discriminate between two enantiomers has been reported in type I (Landsteiner and van der Scheer, 1928, 1929) and between two diasteromes in type IV (Subba Rao et al., 1978) allergies.

Cross-Reactivity

Patients sensitive to usnic acid also react to atranorin and to evernic acid, an observation that may be due (Mitchell and Shibata, 1969) to coincident sensitization. An alternative explanation is that hydrolysis of the ester linkage of the depsides would give substituted phenols (A):

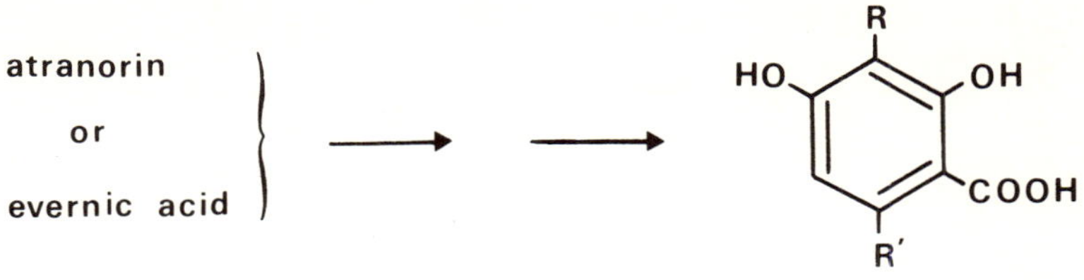

atranorin

or

evernic acid

(A)

The structure of these phenols resembles the structures of compounds (B) and (C) that could be obtained by in vivo oxidative degradation of usnic acid.

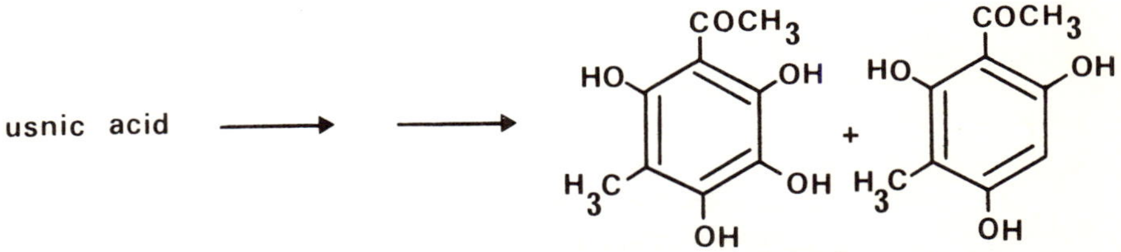

usnic acid

(B)   (C)

Structures (A), (B), and (C) are similar and could yield, by further degradation, a common hapten that would explain the observed cross-reactivity.

The weak cross-reactions to divaricatic acid and perlatolic acid are probably due to the lengthening of the alkyl side chain, from methyl to pentyl, and this is probably a reflection of the size of the combination site on the receptor molecules.

Sphaerophorin should, from the arguments above, give a positive response. This compound was not, however, tested. The results testing with compounds derived from lichenized fungi are summarized in Table 7 and chemical structures of the compounds tested are shown in Fig. 6.

Discussion

The phenomenon of cross-sensitization presents an interesting research and clinical problem. It is unfortunate that, up to now, the fate of haptens in vivo has not been systematically investigated. Consequently, the clinician in investigation of his patients has to rely primarily on his personal experience and on the knowledge of hapten structural similarities in looking for possible cross-reactions. A rationalism of the phenomenon will undoubtedly come

Table 7 Cross-Reactivity among Some Substances Derived from
Lichenized Fungi

Substance	Patch-test results (positive reaction/number of patients tested)
d-Usnic acid	2/3
l-Usnic acid	0/3
l-Dihydrousnic acid	3/4
Atranorin	3/3
Divaricatic acid	1/3
Evernic acid	3/3
Perlatolic acid	1/3 (weak)
Sphaerophorin	not tested

Patients with a history of sensitivity to *d*-usnic acid were patch-tested with
the above compounds suspended in white petroleum jelly U.S.P.

Source: Data from Mitchell and Shibata (1969). © The Williams &
Wilkins Co., Baltimore.

with increased clinical investigations and also with a greater understanding of
the allergen behavior, once the allergen has come in contact with the skin.

However, words of caution must be added in the evaluation of cross-sensitivity reactions. One should be aware of considerations that may cast shadows
on interpretation of the results. For instance, when two compounds are to be
compared, it is important to determine accurately the concentration of each
compound. In addition, it is essential to know if each test substance is pure
or if it is a mixture. Furthermore, it must be established that simultaneous
in vivo tests are independent. These considerations are of major importance
for an unambiguous interpretation of results of patch-testing.

Concentration of Test Substances

The concentration of the test substance is critical: too high a concentration
could lead to an *irritation reaction,* whereas too low a concentration could
give a *false negative* result. It is therefore essential that the substance(s) be
tested at various concentrations. Commercial preparations of haptens sold in

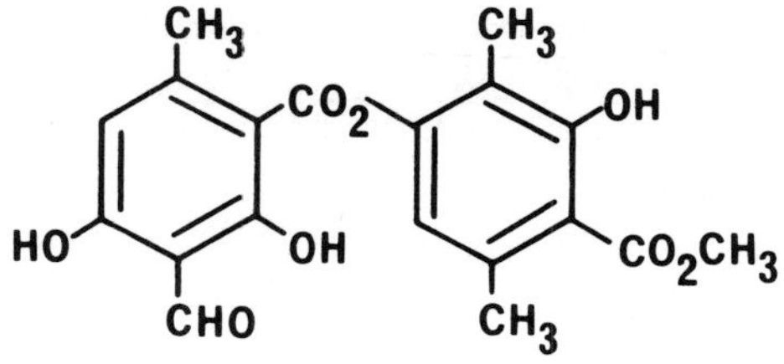

atranorin

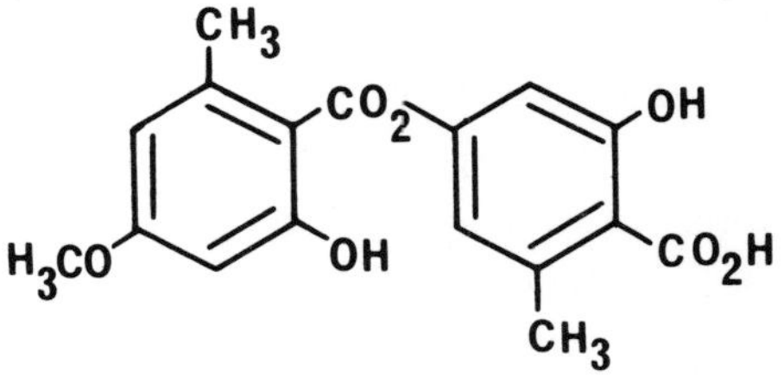

evernic acid

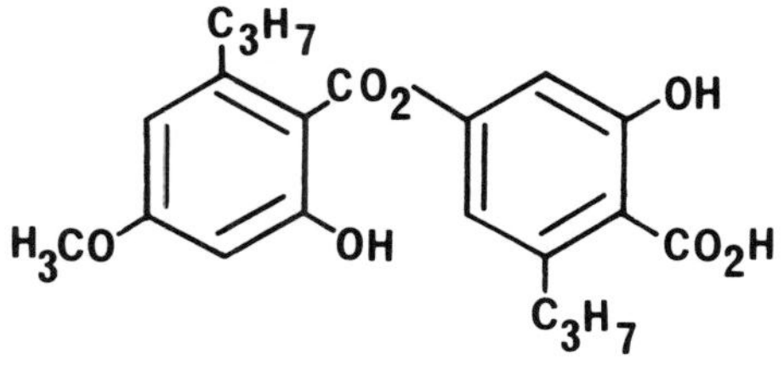

divaricatic acid

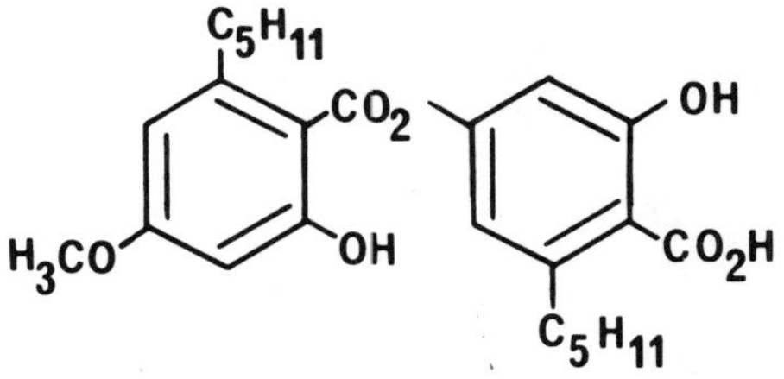

perlatolic acid

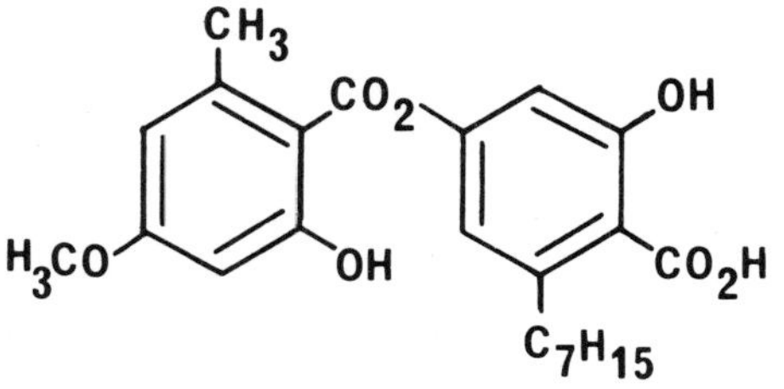

shaerophorin

Figure 6 Chemical structures of the phenolic compounds listed in Table 7.

"test kits" (batteries of allergens) for clinical investigations contain the chemicals dissolved in a solvent or, more often, emulsified in petrolatum jelly. The concentrations of the haptens are usually expressed in percentage, i.e., by weight of hapten in 100 g of "solvent." This does not reflect the situation at the molecular level! For instance, a solution of 0.5% of chromium salt represents in molar equivalents one-fifteenth of a 2% solution of formaldehyde (Benezra et al., 1978). These selected concentrations result from years of experience of dermatologists and are generally satisfactory, although some "flare-up" reactions (spontaneous sensitization) may occur.

Purity of Test Substances

It is of paramount importance to establish that the test substance is pure in order to avoid the possibility of a positive reaction due to the presence of a contaminant (Agrup et al., 1969). A famous example of positive reactions caused by the presence of contaminants is the case of the sodium lauryl ether sulfate (LES) fraction of a dishwashing detergent. This substance was incriminated as the causative agent of an outbreak of contact dermatitis in Scandinavian countries (Ritz et al., 1975). However, the true sensitizer was not LES, but the contaminating chlorosultone and dehydrosultone shown below.

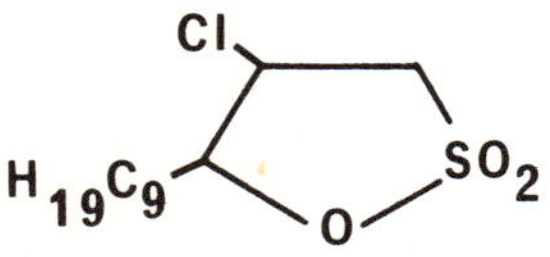

chlorosultone 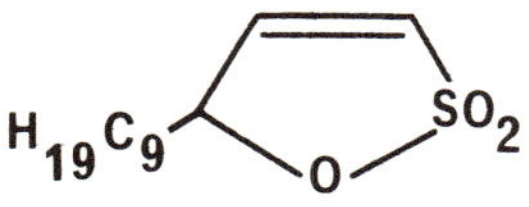   dehydrosultone

$$C_{12}H_{25}SO_3^- \ Na^+$$

sodium lauryl ether sulfate (LES)

The purity of a chemical can be ascertained by a number of physicochemical techniques such as thin-layer or paper chromatography, vapor-phase chromatography, high-performance liquid chromatography (HPLC), melting point (if it is a solid), etc.

The presence of contaminants may also result from instability of the hapten. These contaminants may or may not cause positive reactions. There are also cases where a nonsensitizing substance can, after transformation (degradation, light irradiation, air oxidation, chemical rearrangement, etc.) become contaminated with products which are haptens. This is, for instance, the situation with Δ^3-carene, a constituent of turpentine. Freshly distilled turpentine is nonallergenic, whereas "old" (oxidized) turpentine is a strong sensitizer (Hellerström et al., 1963).

The "Angry Back Syndrome"

Mitchell (1975) has suggested that multiple patchtesting can cause the skin to become hypersensitive. In such a case, a normally negative patch test will be positive because of the concomitant presence of a strong positive test (or tests). This condition, also known as paraallergy (Kligman and Epstein, 1975), has been described as "status eczematicus" or the "angry back syndrome." Hypersensitivity of the skin could thus give false positive patch-test reactions that could obscure and invalidate observations of specific sensitivity or cross-sensitivity to sensitizers.

The influence of skin hypersensitivity in multiple patch tests has been reported by Mitchell (1977). Thirty five outpatients were tested to 28 compounds recommended by the North American Contact Dermatitis Research Group. Patch tests were applied to the upper back. Results were read at day 2 and at day 7 and scored according to the scale of Wilkinson et al. (1970). Twenty three patients who showed one or more +2 reactions and one or more + reactions at day 2 were patch-tested at day 7 to the chemicals that produced positive reactions. Similarly, 12 patients with two or more + reactions were retested on day 7. In both cases, results were read on day 9. On retesting (day 7), 60% of reactions were still positive (as compared with day 2), whereas 42% of the tests were negative. The data were interpreted as supporting the hypothesis that false-positive patch tests are common when concomitant skin tests are performed, i.e., when the tissue is in a state of hyperstimulation.

A further investigation of the angry back syndrome has been recently reported by Bandmann and Agathos (1981). Forty inpatients were patch-tested to a standard series of haptens recommended by the International Contact Dermatitis Research Group, supplemented with common allergens—a total of 26 different compounds. Patch tests were applied to the lower leg. Results were read on day 2, day 3, and day 7. Retesting with substances that elicited positive reactions was carried out by application, in time sequences, of every single substance on the back or by the simultaneous application of three substances on the back and the outer aspects of the upper arms. Successive single tests and groups of three tests were applied at weekly intervals. Results were read at 48 and 72 hr and after 7 days. Results showed that a "loss" of only 8.6% of initially (concomitant testing) positive reactions occurred on retesting.

The data presented by Bandman and Agathos (1981) differ significantly from those reported by Mitchell (1977) and raise several questions regarding the methodology of testing and the real significance of the angry back syndrome. Obviously, these two studies cannot answer these questions, as yet, and further standardized investigations are needed to assess the clinical importance of the mutual influence of concomitant patch tests.

References

Abdou, N. I., and Richter, M. (1970). The role of bone marrow in the immune response. Adv. Immunol. *12*, 201-270.

Abdou, N. I., and Abdou, N. L. (1972). Bone marrow: The bursa equivalent in man. Science *175*, 446-448.

Ada, G. L., Byrt, P., Mandell, T., and Warner, N. (1970). A specific reaction between antigen labelled with radioactive iodine and lymphocyte-like cells from normal, tolerant and immunized mice or rats, in *Developmental Aspects of Antibody Formation and Structure.* Sterzl, J., and Riha, I., eds. Academic Press, New York, pp. 503-516.

Agrup, G., Fregert, S., and Övrum, P. (1969). Importance of pure chemicals in investigations of cross-sensitivity. Acta Dermato-Venereol. *49*, 417-421.

Alkan, S. S., Williams, E. B., Nilecki, D. E., and Goodman, J. W. (1972). Antigen recognition and the immune response. Humoral and cellular immune responses to small, mono- and bifunctional antigen molecules. J. Exp. Med. *135*, 1228-1246.

Archer, O. K., Sutherland, D. E. R., and Good, R. A. (1963). Appendix of the rabbit: A homologue of the bursa in the chicken? Nature *200*, 337-339.

Arnon, R., and Sela, M. (1960). Studies on the chemical basis of the antigenicity of proteins. Biochem. J. *75*, 103-109.

Asherson, G. L., and Ptak, W. (1968). Contact and delayed hypersensitivity in the mouse. I. Active sensitization and passive transfer. Immunology *15*, 405-416.

Astor, S. H., Spitler, L. E., Frick, O. L., and Fudenberg, H. H. (1973). Human leukocyte migration inhibition in agarose using four antigens: Correlation with skin reactivity. J. Immunol. *110*, 1174-1179.

Atassi, M. Z. (1975). Antigenic structure of myoglobin: The complete immunochemical anatomy of a protein and conclusions relating to antigenic structures of proteins. Immunochemistry *12*, 423-438.

Bach, J.-F., Müller, J. Y., and Dardenne, M. (1970). In vivo specific antigen recognition by rosette forming cells. Nature *227*, 1251-1252.

Bach, J.-F. (1973). Evaluation of T-cells and thymic serum factors in man using the rosette technique. Transplant. Rev. *16*, 196-217.

Bach, J. F., and Carnaud, C. (1976). Thymic factors. Progr. Allergy *21*, 342-408.

Bach, J.-F., Dardenne, M., and Pleau, J.-M. (1977). Biochemical characterisation of a serum thymic factor. Nature *266*, 55-57.

Baer, R. L., Serri, F., and Kinman, D. (1952). Attempts at passive transfer of allergic eczematous sensitivity in man by means of white cell suspensions. J. Invest. Derm. *19*, 217-225.

Baer, R. L., and Sulzberger, M. B. (1952). Attempts at passive transfer of allergic eczematous sensitivity in man. J. Invest. Derm. *18*, 53-59.

Baer, R. L. (1954). Cross-sensitization phenomena, in *Modern Trends In Dermatology*, Second series. MacKenna, R. M. B., ed. Butterworths, London, pp. 232-258.

Baer, H., Watkins, R. C., and Bowser, R. T. (1966). Delayed contact sensitivity to catechols and resorcinols. The relationship of structure and immunization procedure to sensitizing capacity. Immunochemistry *3*, 479-485.

Baer, H., Dawson, C. R., and Kurtz, F. (1968). Delayed contact sensitivity to catechols. IV. Sterochemical conformation of the antigenic determinant. J. Immunol. *101*, 1243-1247.

Baer, H., Dawson, C. R., Byck, J. S., and Kurtz, A. P. (1970). The immunochemistry of immune tolerance. II. The relationship of chemical structure to the induction of immune tolerance to catechols. J. Immunol. *104*, 178-184.

Baer, R. L. (1973). Allergic contact sensitization to iron. J. Allergy Clin. Immunol. *51*, 35-38.

Bain, B., Vas, M. R., and Lowenstein, L. (1964). The development of large immature mononuclear cells in mixed leukocyte cultures. Blood *23*, 108-116.

Bandmann, H.-J., and Agathos, M. (1981). New results and some remarks to the "angry back syndrome." Contact Dermatitis *7*, 23-26.

Basten, A., Miller, J. F. A. P., Sprent, J., and Pye, J. (1972a). A receptor for antibody on B lymphocytes. I. Method of detection and functional significance. J. Exp. Med. *135,* 610-626.

Basten, A., Warner, N. L., and Mandell, T. (1972b). A receptor for antibody on B lymphocytes. II. Immunochemical and electron microscopy characteristics. J. Exp. Med. *135,* 627-642.

Bauer, J. A., and Stone, S. H. (1961). Isologous and homologous lymphoid transplant. I. The transfer of tuberculin hypersensitivity in inbred guinea pigs. J. Immunol. *86,* 177-189.

Bauminger, S., Schechter, I., and Sela, M. (1967). Specificity of immunological tolerance to poly-DL-alanyl proteins. Immunochemistry *4,* 169-181.

Bauminger, S., and Sela, M. (1969). Specificity of immunological tolerance to synthetic polypeptides. Israel J. Med. Sci. *5,* 177-184.

Benacerraf, B., and Gell, P. G. H. (1959a). Studies on hypersensitivity. I. Delayed and Arthus-type skin reactivity to protein conjugates in guinea pigs. Immunology *2,* 53-63.

Benacerraf, B., and Gell, P. G. H. (1959b). Studies on hypersensitivity. III. The relation between delayed reactivity to the picryl group of conjugates and contact sensitivity. Immunology *2,* 219-229.

Benacerraf, B., and Levine, B. B. (1962). Immunological specificity of delayed and immediate hypersensitivity reactions. J. Exp. Med. *115,* 1023-1036.

Benacerraf, B., and Dord, M. E. (1974). Genetic control of specific immune response, in *Progress in Immunology,* II, Volume 2. Brent, L., and Holborow, J., eds. North-Holland Publishing Co., Amsterdam, pp. 181-190.

Ben-Efraim, S., and Liacopoulos, P. (1967). Inhibition, no-effect or enhancement of immune response following injection of mixtures of immunogenic and non-immunogenic synthetic polypeptides. Immunology *12,* 517-524.

Ben-Efraim, S., Fuchs, S., and Sela, M. (1967). Differences in immune response to synthetic antigens in two inbred strains of guinea pigs. Immunology *12,* 573-581.

Benezra, C., Andanson, J., Chabeau, C., Ducombs, G., Foussereau, J., Lachapelle, J. M., Lacroix, M., and Martin, P. (1978). Concentrations of patch test allergens: Are we comparing the same thing? Contact Dermatitis *4,* 103-105.

Bennett, B., and Bloom, B. R. (1968). Reactions in vivo and in vitro produced by a soluble substance associated with delayed-type hypersensitivity. Proc. Natl. Acad. Sci. U.S. *59,* 756-762.

Bianco, C., Patrick, R., and Nussenzweig, V. (1970). A population of lymphocytes bearing a membrane receptor for antigen-antibody-complement complexes. J. Exp. Med. *132,* 702-720.

Biberfeld, G. (1973). Macrophage migration inhibition in response to experimental mycoplasma pneumoniae infection in the hamster. J. Immunol. *110*, 1146-1150.

Blanden, R. V. (1974). T-cell response to viral and bacterial infection. Transplant. Rev. *19*, 56-88.

Bloch, B. (1911). Experimentelle Studien über das Wesen der Jodoformidiosynkrasie. Z. fur Exper. Path. Ther. *9*, 509-538.

Bloch, B. (1924). Pathogenese. Arch. Derm. Syph. (Berlin) *145*, 34-82.

Bloch, B., and Steiner-Wourlisch, A. (1926). Die willkurliche Erzeugung der Primeluberemfindlichkeit beim Menschen und ihre Bedeutung für das Idiosyndrasieproblem. Arch. Derm. Syph. *152*, 283-303.

Bloch, B., and Steiner-Wourlisch, A. (1930). Die Sensibilisierung des Meerschweinchens gegen Primeln. Arch. Dermatol. Syph. *162*, 349-378.

Blomgren, H., Takasugi, M., and Friberg, S. (1970). Specific cytotoxicity by sensitized mouse thymus cells on tissue culture target cells. Cell. Immunol. *1*, 616-631.

Bloom, B. R., and Bennett, B. (1966). Mechanism of a reaction in vitro associated with delayed-type hypersensitivity. Science *153*, 80-82.

Bloom, B. R., and Bennett, B. (1969). On the relationship of migration inhibitory factor (MIF) to delayed-type hypersensitivity reactions, in *Cellular Recognition* (4th developmental workshop, Sanibel, 1968). Smith, R. T. and Good, R. A., eds. Appleton-Century-Crofts, New York, pp. 229-234.

Bloom, B. R., Bennett, B., Cettgen, H. F., McLean, E. P., and Old, L. J. (1969). Demonstration of delayed hypersensitivity to soluble antigens of chemically-induced tumors by inhibition of macrophage migration. Proc. Natl. Acad. Sci. U.S. *64*, 1176-1180.

Bloom, B. R., and Bennett, B. (1970). Relation of the migration inhibitory factor (MIF) to delayed-type hypersensitivity reactions. Ann. N.Y. Acad. Sci. *169*, 258-265.

Bloom, B. R., and Jimenez, L. (1970). Migration inhibitory factor and the cellular basis of delayed-type hypersensitivity reactions. Amer. J. Path. *60*, 453-465.

Bloom, B. R. (1971). In vitro approaches to the mechanism of cell-mediated immune reactions. Adv. Immunol. *13*, 101-208.

Bloom, B. R., and Bennett, B. (1971). The assay of inhibition of macrophage migration and the production of migration inhibitory factor (MIF) and skin reactive factor (SRF) in the guinea pig, in *In Vitro Methods in Cell-Mediated Immunity*. Bloom, B. R. and Glade, P. R., eds. Academic Press, New York, pp. 235-248.

Bloom, B. R., and Glade, P. R. (1971). *In Vitro Methods in Cell-Mediated Immunity*. Academic Press, New York.

Borek, F., and Stupp, Y. (1965). Specificity of delayed reactions to hapten-polypeptide conjugates. Immunochemistry 2, 323-328.

Borek, F. (1968). Delayed-type hypersensitivity to synthetic antigens. Curr. Topics Microbiol. Immunol. 43, 126-161.

Borel, Y., and David, J. R. (1970). In vitro studies of the suppression of delayed hypersensitivity by the induction of partial tolerance. J. Exp. Med. 131, 603-610.

Boros, D. L., Schwartz, H. J., Powell, A. E., and Warren, K. S. (1973). Delayed hypersensitivity as manifested by granuloma formation, dermal reactivity, macrophage migration inhibition and lymphocyte transformation, induced and elicited in guinea pigs with soluble antigens to Schistoma mansoni eggs. J. Immunol. 110, 1118-1125.

Boyse, E. A., and Old, L. J. (1969). Some aspects of normal and abnormal cell surface genetics. Annu. Rev. Genet. 3, 269-290.

Brahim, F., and Osmond, O. G. (1970). Migration of bone-marrow lymphocytes demonstrated by selective bone marrow labeling with thymidine-^{3}H. Anat. Rec. 168, 139-151.

Brand, A., Gilmour, D. G., and Goldstein, G. (1976). Lymphocyte-differentiating hormone of bursa of Fabricius. Science 193, 319-321.

Bühler, E. V., and Griffith, F. (1975). Experimental skin sensitisation in the guinea pig and man, in Animal Models in Dermatology, Maibach, H., ed. Churchill Livingstone, Edinburgh, Scotland, pp. 56-66.

Byck, J. S., and Dawson, C. R. (1968). Assay of protein-quinone coupling involving compounds structurally related to the active principle of poison ivy. Anal. Biochem. 25, 123-135.

Camm, E. L., Mitchell, J. C., McMaster, W. R., and Towers, G. H. N. (1975). Subcellular fractions from dermis and epidermis in contact sensitization of guinea pigs to 1-chloro-2,4-dinitrobenzene. Int. Arch. Allergy Appl. Immunol. 48, 276-286.

Cerottini, J. C., Nordin, A. A., and Brunner, K. T. (1970). Specific in vitro cytotoxicity of thymus-derived lymphocytes sensitized to alloantigens. Nature 228, 1308-1309.

Cerottini, J. C., and Brunner, K. T. (1974). Cell-mediated cytotoxicity allograft rejection and tumor immunity. Adv. Immunol. 18, 67-132.

Chase, M. W. (1945). The cellular transfer of cutaneous hypersensitivity to tuberculin. Proc. Soc. Exp. Biol. Med. 59, 134-135.

Chase, M. W. (1954). Experimental sensitization with particular reference to picryl chloride. Int. Arch. Allergy Appl. Immunol. 5, 163-191.

Chase, M. W. (1966). Hypersensitivity to simple chemicals. The Harvey Lectures 61, 169-203.

Cheers, C., Breitner, J. C. S., Little, M., and Miller, J. F. A. P. (1971). Cooperation between carrier-reactive and hapten-sensitive cells in vitro. Nature New Biol. *232*, 248-250.

Chilgren, B. A., Neuwissen, H. J., Quie, P. G., and Hong, R. (1967). Chronic mucocutaneous candidiasis, deficiency of delayed hypersensitivity and selective local antibody defect. Lancet *ii*, 688-693.

Claman, H. N., and Chaperon, E. A. (1969). Immunologic complementation between thymus and marrow cells. A model for the two-cell theory of immunocompetence. Transpl. Rev. *1*, 92-113.

Cline, M. J., and Sweet, V. C. (1968). The interaction of human monocytes and lymphocytes. J. Exp. Med. *128*, 1309-1325.

Cohen, H. A. (1966). Carrier specificity of tuberculin-type reaction to tri-valent chromium. Arch. Derm. *93*, 34-40.

Collotti, C., and Leskowitz, S. (1970). The role of immunogenicity in the induction of tolerance with conjugates of arsanilic acid. J. Exp. Med. *131*, 571-582.

Coombs, R. R. A., and Gell, P. G. H. (1964). The classification of allergic re-actions underlying diseases, in *Clinical Aspects of Immunology*, Second edition. Gell, P. G. H. and Coombs, R. R. A., eds. Blackwell, Oxford, pp. 317-337.

Cooper, M. D., Perey, D. Y., McKneally, M. F., Gabrielsen, A. E., Sutherland, D. E. R., and Good, R. A. (1966). A mammalian equivalent of the avian bursa of Fabricius. Lancet *i*, 1388-1391.

Cooper, M. D., Gabrielsen, A. E., and Good, R. A. (1967). Role of the thy-mus and other central lymphoid tissues in immunological diseases. Ann. Rev. Med. *18*, 113-138.

Cooper, M. D., Gabrielsen, A. E., and Good, R. A. (1968). Central and periph-eral lymphoid tissues in immunologic processes and human diseases in lymph and the lymphatic system, in *Proceedings of the Conference on Lymph and the lymphatic System.* Mayerson, H. D. ed. C. C. Thomas, Springfield, pp. 276-305.

Cooper, M. D., Keightley, R. G., Wu, L. F., and Lawton, A. R. (1973). De-velopmental defects of T and B cell lines in humans. Transpl. Ref. *16*, 51-84.

Coulaud, E. (1935). Caractères de l'état allergique observé chez les animaux de laboratoires après injections de bacilles de Koch enrobés dans la parraf-fine. Compt. Red. Soc. Biol. *119*, 368-369.

Cowling, D. C., Quaglino, D., and Davidson, E. (1963). Changes induced by tuberculin in leukocyte cultures. Lancet *ii*, 1091-1094.

Curtis, J. E., and Hersh, E. M. (1973). Cellular immunity in man: Correlation of leukocyte migration inhibition factor formation and delayed hypersensitivity. Cell. Immunol. *8*, 55-61.

David, J. R., Al-Askari, S., Lawrence, H. S., and Thomas, L. (1964a). Delayed hypersensitivity in vitro. I. The specificity of inhibition of cell migration of antigens. J. Immunol. *93*, 264-273.

David, J. R., Lawrence, H. S., and Thomas, L. (1964b). Delayed hypersensitivity in vitro. II. Effect of sensitive cells on normal cells in the presence of antigen. J. Immunol. *93*, 274-278.

David, J. R., Lawrence, H. S., and Thomas, L. (1964c). Delayed hypersensitivity in vitro. III. The specificity of hapten-protein conjugates in the inhibition of cell migration. J. Immunol. *93*, 279-282.

David, J. R. (1966). Delayed hypersensitivity in vitro. Its mediation by cell-free substances formed by lymphoid cell-antigen interaction. Proc. Natl. Acad. Sci. U.S. *56*, 72-77.

David, J. R., and Schlossman, S. F. (1968). Immunochemical studies on the specificity of cellular hypersensitivity. The in vitro inhibition of peritoneal exudate cell migration by chemically defined antigens. J. Exp. Med. *128*, 1451-1459.

David, J. R., and David, R. (1971). Assay for inhibition of macrophage migration, in *In Vitro Methods in Cell-Mediated Immunity*. Bloom, B. R., and Glade, P. R., eds. Academic Press, New York, pp. 249-261.

David, J. R., and David, R. R. (1972). Cellular hypersensitivity and immunity. Inhibition of macrophage migration and the lymphocyte mediators. Progr. Allergy *16*, 300-449.

Davies, A. J. S. (1969). The thymus and the cellular basis of immunity. Transplant Rev. *1*, 43, 91.

Dawson, C. R. (1956). The chemistry of poison ivy. Annals N.Y. Acad. Sci. *18*, 427-443.

Delacretaz, J., and Geiser, J. P. (1960). Nouvelles recherches sur les facteurs allergiques dans l'eczéma au ciment. Symp. Dermatologurum, Pragae *1*, 245-249.

Dickler, H. B., and Kunkel, H. G. (1972). Interaction of aggregated γ-globulin with B lymphocytes. J. Exp. Med. *136*, 191-196.

Dienes, L. (1928). Further observations concerning the sensitization of tuberculous guinea pigs. J. Immunol. *15*, 153-174.

Draize, J. H. (1955). Dermal Toxicity. Food Drug Cosmet. Law J. *10*, 722-732.

Dumonde, D. C., Wolstencroft, R. A., Panayi, G. S., Matthew, M., Morlew, J., and Howson, W. T. (1969). Lymphokines: Non-antibody mediators of cellular immunity generated by lymphocyte activation. Nature *224*, 38-43.

Dupuis, G., Mitchell, J. C., and Towers, G. H. N. (1974). Reaction of alantolactone, an allergenic sesquiterpene lactone, with some amino acids. Result-
ant loss of immunologic reactivity. Can. J. Biochem. *52*, 575-581.

Dupuis, G., and Brisson, J. (1976). Toxic effect of alantolactone and dihydroalantolactone in in vitro cultures of leukocytes. Chemico-biol. Interact. *15*,
205-217.

Dupuis, G. (1979). Studies on poison ivy. In vitro lymphocyte transformation
by urushiol-protein conjugates. Brit. J. Derm. *101*, 617-624.

Dupuis, G., Benezra, C., Schlewer, G., and Stampf, J. L. (1980). Allergic contact dermatitis to α-methylene-γ-butyrolactones. Preparation of alantolactone-
skin protein conjugates and induction of contact sensitivity in the guinea pig
by an alantolactone-skin protein conjugate. Molecular Immunol. *17*, 1045-
1051.

Dupuy, J. M., Perey, D. Y. E., and Good, R. A. (1969). Passive transfer, with
plasma, of delayed allergy in guinea pigs. Lancet *i*, 551-553.

Dupuy, J. M., Perey, D. Y. E., and Good, R. A. (1970a). Transfer of skin
homograft immunity with a plasma factor. J. Immunol. *104*, 1384-1387.

Dupuy, J. M., Kalpaktosoglu, P., and Good, R. A. (1970b). Transfer with a
plasma fraction of delayed hypersensitivity to PPD in guinea pigs. J. Immunol. *104*, 1384-1387.

Dupuy, J. M., and Good, R. A. (1970). Role of lymphoid cells in passive transfer with plasma of delayed hypersensitivity in guinea pigs. J. Immunol. *105*,
1111-1115.

Dupuy, J. M., and Good, R. A. (1971). Passive transfer of delayed hypersensitivity in guinea pigs. Role of conventional antibody and antigen. J. Immunol. *106*, 528-535.

Eden, A., Bianco, C., and Nussenzweig, V. (1971). A population of lymphocytes bearing a membrane receptor for antigen-antibody-complement complexes. II. Specific isolation. Cell Immunol. *2*, 658-669.

Eisen, H. N., Orris, L., and Belman, S. (1952). Elicitation of delayed allergic
skin reaction with haptens: The dependence of elicitation on hapten combination with protein. J. Exp. Med. *95*, 473-487.

Eisen, H. N., and Belman, S. (1953). Studies of hypersensitivity to low molecular weight substances. II. Reactions of some allergenic substituted dinitro-
benzenes with cysteine or cystine of skin proteins. J. Exp. Med. *98*, 533-549.

Eisen, H. N., and Tabachnick, M. (1958). Elicitation of allergic contact dermatitis in the guinea pig. The distribution of bound dinitrobenzene groups
within the skin and quantitative determination of the extent of combination
of 2,4-dinitrochlorobenzene with epidermal protein in vivo. J. Exp. Med.
108, 773-796.

Eisen, H. N., Kern, M., Newton, W. J., and Helmreich, E. (1959). A study of the distribution of 2,4-dinitrobenzene sensitizers between isolated lymph node cells and extracellular medium in reaction to induction of contact skin sensitivity. J. Exp. Med. *110*, 187-206.

Eisen, H. N. (1959). Hypersensitivity to simple chemicals, in *Cellular and Humoral Aspects of the Hypersensitive State.* Lawrence, H. S., ed. Hoeber-Harper, New York, pp. 89-122.

Eisen, H. N. (1964). Preparation of purified anti-2,4-dinitrophenyl antibodies. Methods Med. Res. *10*, 94-102.

Emmet, E. A., and Suskind, R. R. (1973). Allergic contact sensitization to the toluic acids. J. Invest. Derm. *61*, 282-285.

Epstein, W. L., and Kligman, A. M. (1957). Transfer of allergic contact-type delayed sensitivity in man. J. Invest. Derm. *28*, 291-304.

Fahr, H., Noster, U., and Schulz, K. H. (1976). Comparison of guinea pig sensitization methods. Contact Dermatitis *2*, 335-339.

Feinstone, S. M., Beachey, E. H., and Rytel, M. W. (1969). Induction of delayed hypersensitivity to influenza and mumps viruses in mice. J. Immunol. *103*, 844-849.

Feldman, M., and Palmer, J. (1971). The requirement for macrophages in the secondary immune response to antigens of small and large size. Immunology *21*, 685-699.

Fieser, C., and Fieser, M. (1967). *Reagents for Organic Synthesis,* Volume 1. John Wiley & Sons, New York.

Fisher, A. A. (1973). *Contact Dermatitis,* Second edition. Lea and Febiger, Philadelphia.

Ford, W. L. (1973). The cellular basis of immunes responses. in *Defence and Recognition,* MTP International Review of Science, Biochemistry series one, Volume 10. Porter, R. R., ed. Butterworths, London, pp. 65-102.

Foussereau, J. (1963). La pipérazine, un allergène de contact chez le personnel soignant. Rev. franc. Allergie *3*, 236-243.

Foussereau, J., and Benezra, C. (1967). Données nouvelles sur l'allergie de groupe à la pipérazine. Bull. Soc. franc. Derm. Syph. *74*, 45-48.

Foussereau, J., Mme Petitjean, L., Heid, E., and Basset, A. (1969). Intérêt du test à la primine dans l'eczéma de contact à la primevère. Bull. Soc. franc. Derm. Syph. *76*, 458-461.

Foussereau, J., and Benezra, C. (1970). *Les Eczémas Allergiques Profession-nels.* Masson et Cie, Paris.

Foussereau, J., and Benezra, C., and Maibach, H. I. (1982). Occupational Contact Dermatitis: Clinical and Chemical Aspects, Monksgaard, Copenhagen.

Fregert, S., and Rorsman, H. (1960). Hypersensitivity to diethylstilbestrol, hexestrol, bisphenol A, p-benzylphenol, hydroquinone-monobenzyl ether, and *p*-hydroxybenzoic acid benzyl ester. Acta Dermato-Venereol. *40,* 206-219.

Fregert, S., Hjorth, N., and Schulz, K. H. (1968). Patch testing with synthetic primin in persons sensitive to *Primula obconica.* Arch. Derm. *98,* 144-147.

Freund, J. (1926). On the role of the reticulo-endothelial system in tuberculin hypersensitiveness. J. Immunol. *11,* 383-391.

Freund, J., Casals, J., and Hosmer, E. P. (1938). Sensitization and antibody formation after injections of tubercule bacilli and paraffin oil. Proc. Soc. Exp. Biol. Med. *37,* 509-513.

Freund, J., and McDermott, K. (1942). Sensitization to horse serum by means of adjuvants. Proc. Soc. Exp. Biol. Med. *49,* 548-553.

Frey, J. R., and Wenk, P. (1957). Experimental studies on the pathogens of contact eczema in the guinea pig. Int. Arch. Allergy Appl. Immunol. *11,* 81-100.

Frey, J. R., and Geleick, H. (1959). Experimentelles Kontaktezkem durch Dinitrochlorbenzol an Ratten und Kaninchen. Dermatologia *119,* 294-300.

Friend, J. V., and Lane, M. (1973). In vitro studies of contact hypersensitivity. The effect of the haptens 2,4-dinitrochlorobenzene (DNCB) and 2,4-dinitrofluorobenzene (DNFB) and of hapten-protein conjugates on the migration of guinea pig peritoneal exudate cells. Immunology *25,* 869-874.

Fuchs, C. H. (1840). Die krankhaften Veranderungen der Haut-und ihre Anhänge, Göttingen Dieterichsche Buchhandlung *1,* 87-98.

Geczy, A. F., and Baumgarten, A. (1970). Lymphocyte transformation in contact sensitivity. Immunology *19,* 189-203.

Gell, P. G. H., Harington, C. R., and Rivers, R. P. (1946). The antigenic function of simple chemical compounds: Production of precipitins in rabbits. Brit. J. Exp. Path. *27,* 267-386.

Gell, P. G. H., and Hinde, I. T. (1951). The histology of the tuberculin reaction and its modification by cortisone. Brit. J. Exp. Path. *32,* 516-529.

Gell, P. G. H., and Benacerraf, B. (1961). Studies on hypersensitivity. IV. The relationship between contact and delayed sensitivity. A study on the specificity of cellular immune reaction. J. Exp. Med. *113,* 571-585.

Gell, P. G. H., and Silverstein, A. M. (1962). Delayed hypersensitivity to hapten-protein conjugates. I. The effect of carrier protein and site of attachment to hapten. J. Exp. Med. *115,* 1037-1051.

George, M., and Vaughan, J. H. (1962). In vitro cell migration as a model for delayed hypersensitivity. Proc. Soc. Exp. Biol. Med. *111,* 514-521.

Glick, D. M., Goren, H. J., and Barnard, E. A. (1967). Concurrent bromoacetate reaction at histidine and methonine residues in ribonuclease. Biochem. J. *102,* 7C-10C.

Godfrey, H. P., Baer, H., and Chaparas, S. D. (1969). Inhibition of macrophage migration by a skin-reactive polysaccharide from BCG-culture filtrates. J. Immunol. *102,* 1466-1473.

Godfrey, H. P., Baer, H., and Watkins, R. C. (1971). Delayed hypersensitivity to catechols. V. Absorption and distribution of substances related to poison ivy extracts and their relation to the induction of sensitization and tolerance. J. Immunol. *106,* 91-102.

Goldstein, G. (1974). Isolation of bovine thymin: A polypeptide hormone of the thymus. Nature *247,* 11-14.

Goldstein, A. L., Low, T. L. K., McAdoo, M., McClure, J., Thurman, G. B., Rossio, J., Lai, C. Y., Chang, D., Wang, S.-S., Harvey, C., Ramel, A. H., and Meienhofer, J. (1977). Thymosin α_1: Isolation and sequence analysis of an immunologically active thymic polypeptide. Proc. Natl. Acad. Sci. U.S. *74,* 725-729.

Good, R. A., Varco, R. L., Aust, J. G., and Zak, S. J. (1957). Transplantation studies in patients with agammaglobulinemia. Ann. N.Y. Acad. Sci. *64,* 882-928.

Good, R. A., Gabrielsen, A. E., Peterson, R. D. A., Finstad, J., and Cooper, M. D. (1966). The development of the central and peripheral lymphoid tissue: Ontogenetic and phylogenetic considerations, in *The Thymus, Experimental and Clinical Studies.* Wolstenholme, G. W. and Porter, R., eds. Ciba Foundation Symposium. Little, Brown and Co., Boston, pp. 181-213.

Goodman, M. H. (1941). Cutaneous hypersensitivity to the procaine anesthetics. Correlation of hypersensitivity with chemical structure. J. Invest. Derm. *2,* 53-66.

Gordon, J., and MacLean, L. D. (1965). A lymphocyte-stimulating factor produced in vitro. Nature *208,* 795-796.

Gordon, J. (1968). Role of monocytes in the mixed leukocyte culture reaction. Proc. Soc. Exp. Biol. Med. *127,* 30-33.

Gotoff, S. P., and Vizral, I. F. (1972). The macrophage aggregation assay for delayed hypersensitivity: Development of the response, role of the macrophage and the independence of humoral antibody. Cell. Immunol. *3,* 53-61.

Granger, G. A., and Williams, T. W. (1968). Lymphocyte cytotoxicity in vitro. Activation and release of a cytotoxic factor. Nature *218,* 1253-1254.

Grasbeck, R., Nordman, C. T., and de la Chapelle, A. (1964). The leukocyte-mitogenic effect of serum from rabbits immunized with human leukocytes. Acta Med. Scand. Suppl. *412,* 39-47.

Greaves, M. F. (1970). Biological effects of anti-immunoglobulins: Evidence for immunoglobulin receptors on T and B lymphocytes. Transplant. Rev. *5,* 45-75.

Greaves, M. F., and Möller, E. (1970a). The origin and significance of rosette forming cells in the response of mice to sheep erythrocytes, in *Developmental Aspects of Antibody Formation and Structure*. Sterzl, J. and Riha, I., eds. Academic Press, New York, pp. 627-633.

Greaves, M. F., and Möller, E. (1970b). Studies on antigen binding cells. I. The origin of reactive cells. Cell. Immunol. *1*, 372-385.

Green, I., Paul, W. E., and Benacerraf, B. (1966). The behavior of hapten-poly-L-Lysine conjugates as complete antigens in genetic responders and as haptens in non-responder guinea pigs. J. Exp. Med. *123*, 859-879.

Green, J. A., Cooperband, S. E., and Kibrick, S. (1969). Immune specific induction of interferon production in cultures of human blood lymphocytes. Science *164*, 1415-1417.

Green, W. C., Wedner, H. J., and Parker, C. W. (1976). Calcium ionophore A23187 and lymphocyte activation, in *Leukocyte Membrane Determinants Regulating Immune Reactivity*. Eijswoogel, V.P., Roos, D., and Zeijlmaker, W. P., eds. Academic Press, New York, p. 129.

Greenstein, J. P., and Winitz, M. (1961). *Chemistry of the Amino Acids*. John Wiley & Sons, New York.

Gross, E., and Witkop, B. (1962). Nonenzymatic cleavage of peptide bonds: The methionine residues in bovine pancreatic ribonuclease. J. Biol. Chem. *237*, 1856-1860.

Gross, P. R., Katz, S. A., and Mamitz, M. H. (1968). Sensitization of guinea pigs to chromium salts. J. Invest. Derm. *50*, 424-427.

Hall, J., and Smith, M. E. (1971). Studies on the afferent and efferent lymph of the lymph node draining the site of application of fluorodinitrobenzene (FDNB). Immunology *21*, 69-79.

Hamilton, L. D., and Chase, M. W. (1962). Labelled cells in the cellular transfer of delayed hypersensitivity in allergic eczema. Fed. Proc. *21*, 40.

Hanna, N., Ferraresi, R. W., and Leskowitz, S. (1973). In vitro correlates of hapten-specific delayed hypersensitivity. Cell. Immunol. *8*, 155-161.

Hanna, N., and Leskowitz, S. (1973a). Structural requirements for in vivo and in vitro immunogenicity in hapten-specific delayed hypersensitivity. Cell. Immunol. *7*, 189-197.

Hanna, N., and Leskowitz, S. (1973b). Structural requirements for antigen in lymphocyte stimulation, in *Proceeding of the Seventh Leukocyte Culture Conference*. Daguillard, F., ed. Academic Press, New York, pp. 217-229.

Harber, L. E., and Baer, R. L. (1961). Attempts to transfer eczematous contact-type allergy with whole blood transfusions. J. Invest. Derm. *36*, 55-58.

Hartwell, J. L., and Abbott, B. (1969). Antineoplastic principles in plants; recent developments in the field. Adv. Pharmacol. Chemother. *7*, 117-209.

Hashimoto, K. (1971). Langerhans cell granule. An endocytotic organelle. Arch. Dermatol. *104*, 148-160.

Hausen, B. (1973). *Holzarten mit gesundheitschadigenden Inhaltstoffen.* D.R.W.-Verlags-GmbH, Stuttgart.

Haxthausen, H. (1947). Studies on the role of the lymphocyte as transmitters of the hypersensitiveness in allergic eczema. Acta Dermato-Venereol. *27*, 275-286.

Haxthausen, H. (1951). Passive transmission of dinitrochlorobenzene allergy with white blood cells from sensitized guinea pigs. Acta Dermato-Venereol. *31*, 656-665.

Haxthausen, H. (1953). Attempts on passive local sensitization by intracutaneous injection of cells from freshly excised lymph nodes of eczema allergics. J. Invest. Derm. *21*, 237-241.

Hebra, F. (1869). *Traité des Maladies de la Peau,* Volume 1. Masson et Cie, Paris, pp. 493-496, 541-542.

Heilman, D. H., and McFarland, W. (1966a). Inhibition of tuberculin-induced mitogenesis in cultures of lymphocytes from tuberculous donors. Int. Arch. Allergy Appl. Immunol. *30*, 58-66.

Heilman, D. H., and McFarland, W. (1966b). Mitogenic activity of bacterial fractions in lymphocyte cultures. 1. Purified protein derivative and polysaccharides of tuberculin. J. Immunol. *96*, 988-991.

Hellerström, S., Lodin, A., Rajka, G., Swedin, B., and Widmark, G. (1963). Sensitization of pigs with 3-carene. Acta Dermato-Venereol. *43*, 311-321.

Henney, C. S. (1973). On the mechanism of T cell-mediated cytolysis. Transplant. Rev. *17*, 37-70.

Herman, P. S., and Sams Jr., W. M. (1971). Requirement for carrier protein in salicylanilide sensitivity: The migration—inhibition test in contact photoallergy. J. Lab. Clin. Med. *77*, 572-579.

Herman, P. S., and Sams Jr., W. M. (1972). *Soap Photodermatitis. Photosensitivity to Halogenated Salicylanilides.* C. C. Thomas Publishing Co., Springfield, Illinois.

Hersh, E. M., and Harris, J. E. (1968). Macrophage-lymphocyte interaction in the antigen-induced blastogenic response of human peripheral blood leukocytes. J. Immunol. *100*, 1184-1194.

Hirschhorn, K., Schreibman, R. R., Verbo, S., and Gruskin, R. H. (1964). The action of streptolysin S on peripheral lymphocytes of normal subjects and patients with acute rheumatic fever. Proc. Natl. Acad. Sci. U.S. *52*, 1151-1157.

Hjorth, N., and Fregert, S. (1979). Contact Dermatitis, in *Textbook of Dermatology,* Volume One, Third Edition. Rook, A., Wilkinson, D. S. and Ebling, F. J. G., eds. Blackwell Scientific Publication, Oxford, pp. 363-441.

Hoogewerff, S., and van Dorp, W. A. (1879). Über die Oxydation von Chinolin Vermittel Kalium Permanganat. Chem. Ber. *12,* 747-748.

Hungerford, D. A., Donnelly, A. J., Nowell, P. C., and Beck, S. (1959). The chromosome constitution of a human phenotype intersex. Am. J. Hum. Genetics *11,* 215-236.

Huriez, C., Agache, P., Martin, P., Vandamme, G., and Mennecier, M. (1965). Un groupe d'allergènes chimiques fréquemment en cause, les sels d'ammonium quaternaires. Rev. franc. Allergie *5,* 134-142.

Hutchison, F., Raffle, E. J., and Macleod, T. M. (1972). The specificity of lymphocyte transformation in vitro by nickel salts in nickel sensitive subjects. J. Invest. Derm. *58,* 362-365.

Hutchison, F., Macleod, T. M., and Raffle, E. J. (1975). Nickel hypersensitivity. Nickel binding to amino acids and lymphocytes. Brit. J. Derm. *93,* 557-561.

Inderbitzin, T. (1956). The relationship of lymphocytes, delayed cutaneous allergic reactions and histamine. In. Arch. Allergy Appl. Immunol. *8,* 150-159.

Indgin, S. N., and Inderbitzin, T. M. (1971). An attempt to transfer delayed allergic contact sensitivity to DNCB with plasma. Int. Arch. Allergy Appl. Immunol. *41,* 868-872.

Itakura, K., Hutton, J. J., Boyse, E. A., and Old, L. J. (1972). Genetic linkage relationships of loci specifying differentiation alloantigens in the mouse. Transplantation *13,* 239-243.

Jadassohn, J. (1895). Zur Kenntnis Medicamentösen Dermatosen. Vehr. Deutsch. Derm. Ges. *5,* 103.

Jadassohn, J. (1896). Zur Kenntnis Arzneiexantheme. Arch. Derm. Syph. (Berlin) *34,* 103.

Jadassohn, W. (1930). Sensibilisierung der Haut des Meerscheinchens auf Phenylhydrazin. Klin. Wochenschr. *9,* 551.

Jaeger, H., and Pelloni, E. (1950). Test épicutanés aux bichromates, positifs dans l'eczéma au ciment. Dermatologica *100,* 207-216.

James, B. M. (1931). Procaine dermatitis: Report of a case and attempt to determine chemical groups responsible for hypersensitiveness. J. Am. Med. Ass. *97,* 440-442.

James, M. N. G. (1980). An X-ray crystallographic approach to enzyme structure and function. Can. J. Biochem. *58,* 251-271.

Janeway, C. A. (1975a). Cellular cooperation during in vivo antihapten antibody responses. I. The effect of cell number on the response. J. Immunol. *114*, 1394-1401.

Janeway, C. A. (1975b). Cellular cooperation during in vivo anti-hapten antibody responses. I. The effect of in vivo and in vitro X-irradiation on T and B cells. J. Immunol. *114*, 1402-1407.

Jenkins, W. T., and Sizer, I. W. (1959). Glutamic aspartic transaminase. The influence of pH on absorption spectrum and enzymatic activity. J. Biol. Chem. *234*, 1179-1181.

Johnson, R. A., Baer, H., Kirkpatrick, C. H., Dawson, C. R., and Khurana, R. G. (1972). Comparison of the contact allergenicity of the four pentadecylcatechols derived from poison ivy urushiol in human subjects. J. Allergy Clin. Immunol. *49*, 27-35.

Johnston, A. J. M., and Calnan, C. D. (1958). Cement dermatitis. Chemical aspects. Trans. St-John's Hosp. Derm. Soc. *41*, 11-25.

Jung, E. G., Hornke, J., and Hajdu, P. (1968). Photoallergie durch 4-chlor-2-hydroxy-benzosaüre-n-butylamid. Arch. Klin. Exp. Derm. *233*, 287-295.

Kantor, F. S., Odeja, A., and Benacerraf, B. (1963). Studies on artificial antigens. 1. Antigenicity of DNP-polysine and DNP-copolymer of lysine and glutamic acid in guinea pigs. J. Exp. Med. *117*, 55-69.

Kantor, G. L., and Dixon, F. J. (1972). Transfer of experimental allergic orchitis with peritoneal exudate cells. J. Immunol. *108*, 329-338.

Kasakura, S., and Lowenstein, L. (1965). Haematology. A factor stimulating DNA synthesis derived from the medium of leukocyte cultures. Nature *208*, 794-795.

Katz, D. H., and Benaceraff, B. (1972). The regulatory influence of activated T cells on B cell responses to antigen. Adv. Immunol. *15*, 1-94.

Katz, D. H. (1977). *Lymphocyte Differentiation, Recognition and Regulation.* Academic Press, New York.

Kay, K., and Rieke, W. O. (1963). Tuberculin hypersensitivity: Studies with radioactive antigens and mononuclear cells. Science *139*, 487-490.

Keil, H., Wasserman, D., and Dawson, C. R. (1944). The relation of chemical structure in catechol compounds and derivatives to poison ivy hypersensitiveness in man as shown by patch tests. J. Exp. Med. *80*, 275-287.

Kirchheimer, W. F., and Weiser, R. S. (1947). The tuberculin reaction. I. Passive transfer of tuberculin sensitivity with cells of tuberculous guinea pigs. Proc. Soc. Exp. Biol. Med. *66*, 166-172.

Kisken, W. A., and Swenson, N. A. (1969). Unresponsiveness of mixed leukocyte cultures from thymectomized adult dogs. Nature *224*, 76-77.

Kitagawa, I., Yamazoe, Y., Takeda, R., and Yoshioka, I. (1972). Conversion of dihydroalantolactone to eremophilane-type derivatives: A biogenetic-type transformation. Tetrahedron Letters 4843-4846.

Kitagawa, I., Shibuya, H., Yamazoe, Y., Takeno, H., and Yoshioka, I. (1974). Conversion of dihydroalantolactone to tetrahydroligularenolide. A biogenetic-type transformation of eudesmanolide to eremophilanolide. Tetrahedron Letters 111-114.

Klecak, G. (1977). Identification of contact allergens: Predictive tests in animals, in *Dermatotoxicology and Pharmacology. Advances in Modern Toxicology,* Volume 4. Marzulli, F. N. and Maibach, H. I., eds. Hemisphere Publishing Company, Washington, pp. 305-339.

Klecak, G., Geleick, H., and Frey, J. R. (1977). Screening of fragrance materials for allergenicity in the guinea pig. I. Comparison of four testing methods. J. Soc. Cosmet. Chem. *28,* 53-64.

Kligman, A. M. (1958). Poison ivy (*Rhus*) dermatitis. Archiv. Derm. *77,* 149-180.

Kligman, A. M. (1966a). The SLS provocative test in allergic contact sensitization. J. Invest. Derm. *46,* 573-581.

Kligman, A. M. (1966b). The identification of contact allergens by human assay. I. A critique of standard methods. J. Invest. Derm. *47,* 369-374.

Kligman, A. M. (1966c). The identification of contact allergens by human assay. II. Factors influencing the induction and measurement of allergic contact dermatitis. J. Invest. Derm. *47,* 375-392.

Kligman, A. M. (1966d). The identification of contact allergens by human assay. III. The maximization test: A procedure for screening and rating contact sensitizers. J. Invest. Derm. *47,* 393-409.

Kligman, A. M., and Epstein, W. (1975). Updating the maximization test for identifying contact allergens. Contact Dermatitis *1,* 231-239.

Knight, S. C., Newey, B., and Ling, N. R. (1973). Thymus dependence in the rat of lymphocytes responding to stimulation with specific antigen, allogenic lymphocytes and non-specific mitogens. Cytobios *7,* 35-49.

Koch, R. (1890). Weitere Mitteilungen ueber ein heilmittel gegen Tuberkulose. Deutsch. Med. Wschr. *16,* 1029.

Kolb, W. P., and Granger, G. A. (1968). Lymphocyte in vitro cytotoxicity. Characterization of human lymphotoxin. Proc. Natl. Acad. Sci. U.S. *61,* 1250-1255.

Kronman, B. S., Wepsic, H. T., Churchill, W. H., Zbar, B., Borsos, T., and Rapp, H. J. (1969). Tumor-specific antigens detected by inhibition of macrophage migration. Science *165,* 296-297.

Kruger, J., Wsyland, J. S., and Waskman, B. H. (1971). Specificity of delayed responses to hapten-protein conjugates in rats. Immunochem. *8,* 319-323.

Kupchan, S. M., Fessler, D. C., Eakin, M. A., and Giacobbe, T. J. (1970). Reactions of alpha-methylene lactone tumor inhibitors with model biological nucleophiles. Science *168,* 376-378.

Kupchan, S. M., Eakin, M. A., and Thomas, A. M. (1971). Tumor inhibitors.
69. Structure-cytotoxicity of sesquiterpene lactones. J. Med. Chem. *14,*
1147-1152.

Kutney, J. P., and Sanchez, I. H. (1976). Studies in the usnic acid series. I.
The condensation of (-)-usnic acid with aliphatic and aromatic amines.
Can. J. Chem. *54,* 2795-2803.

Landsteiner, K., and Lampl, H. (1918). Ueber di Abhängigkeit der serologi-
schen Spezificität von der chemischen Struktur (Darstellung von Antigenene
mit bekannter chemischer Konstitution des spezifischen Gruppen). XII.
Mitteilung über Antigene. Biochem. Z. *86,* 343-394.

Landsteiner, K., and van der Scheer, J. (1928). Serological differentiation of
steric isomers. J. Exp. Med. *48,* 315-320.

Landsteiner, K., and van der Scheer, J. (1929). Serological differentiation of
steric isomers (antigens containing tartaric acids). Second paper. J. Exp.
Med. *50,* 407-417.

Landsteiner, K., and Jacobs, J. L. (1936). Studies on the sensitization of
animals with simple chemical compounds. III. J. Exp. Med. *64,* 625-639.

Landsteiner, K., and Chase, M. W. (1941). Studies on the sensitization of animals with simple chemical compounds. IX. Skin sensitization induced by
injection of conjugates. J. Exp. Med. *73,* 431-438.

Landsteiner, K., and Chase, M. W. (1942). Experiments on transfer of cutaneous sensitivity to simple compounds. Proc. Soc. Exp. Biol. Med. *49,*
688-690.

Lawrence, H. S. (1949). The cellular transfer of cutaneous hypersensitivity to
tuberculin in man. Proc. Soc. Exp. Biol. Med. *71,* 516-522.

Lawrence, H. S. (1955). The transfer in humans of delayed skin sensitivity to
streptococcal M substance and to tuberculin with leucocytes. J. Clin. Invest. *34,* 219-230.

Lawrence, H. S. (1969). Transfer factor. Adv. Immunol. *11,* 195-266.

Lawrence, H. S. (1972-1973). Transfer factor in cellular immunity. The
Harvey Lectures *68,* 239-350.

Lay, W. H., and Nussenzweig, V. (1968). Receptors for complement on leukocytes. J. Exp. Med. *128,* 991-1007.

Lee, K., Huang, E., Piantodosi, C., Pagano, J. S., and Geissman, T. A. (1971).
Cytotoxicity of sesquiterpene lactones. Cancer Res. *31,* 1649-1654.

Leifer, W., and Steiner, K. (1951). Studies in sensitization to halogenated
hydroxyquinolines and related compounds. J. Invest. Derm. *17,* 233-240.

Leon, M. A., and Takahashi, T. (1970). Stimulation of lymphocytes by
myeloma proteins, in *Proceeding of the Fifth Leukocyte Culture Conference.* Harris, J. E., ed. Academic Press, New York, pp. 299-304.

Leskowitz, S. (1963a). Immunochemical study of antigenic specificity in de-

layed hypersensitivity. II. Delayed hypersensitivity to polytyrosineazo-
benzenearsonate and its suppression by haptens. J. Exp. Med. *117*, 909-
923.

Leskowitz, S. (1963b). Use of oxidized proteins in the examination of immunochemical specificity in delayed hypersensitivity to hapten-protein
conjugates. Nature *199*, 85-86.

Leskowitz, S., Jones, V. E., and Zak, S. J. (1966). Immunochemical study
of antigenic specificity in delayed hypersensitivity. V. Immunization with
monovalent low molecular weight conjugates. J. Exp. Med. *123*, 229-237.

Leskowitz, S., Richerson, H. B., and Schwartz, J. J. (1970). Amino acid contribution to hapten specificity in delayed reaction to arsanilic acid conjugates. Immunochem. *7*, 949-954.

Levine, B. B., Ojeda, A., and Benaceraff, B. (1963). Studies on artificial
antigens. III. The genetic control of the immune response to hapten-poly-
L-lysine conjugates in guinea pigs. J. Exp. Med. *118*, 953-957.

Levis, W. R., Whalen, M. S., and Powell, J. A. (1975). Studies on the contact
sensitization of man with simple chemicals. III. Quantitative relationships
between specific lymphocyte transformation, skin sensitivity, and lymphokine activity in response to dinitrochlorobenzene. J. Invest. Derm. *64*, 100-
104.

Ling, N. R., and Kay, J. E. (1975). *Lymphocyte Stimulation.* American
Elsevier Publishing Co., New York.

Lis, H., and Sharon, N. (1973). The biochemistry of plant lectins (phyto-
hemagglutinins). Ann. Rev. Biochem. *42*, 541-574.

Low, T. L. K., and Goldstein, A. L. (1979). Thymosin and other thymic hormones and their synthetic analogues. Springer Seminars Immunopathol. *2*,
169-186.

Macher, E. (1962a). Die Reaktion der regionaren Lymphknoten beim tier-
experimentellen allergischen Kontaktekzem. I. Makroscopische Untersuchugen. Hautartz, *13*, 18-23.

Macher, E. (1962b). Die Reaktion der regionaren Lymphknoten beim tier-
experimentellen allergischen Kontaktekzem. II. Histologische Untersuch-
ungen. Hautartz *13*, 126-131.

Macher, E. (1962c). Die Reaktion der regionaren Lymphknoten beim tier-
experimentellen allergischen Kontaktekzem. III. Cytologische Untersuch-
ungen. Hautartz *13*, 174-179.

Macher, E., and Chase, M. W. (1969). Studies on the sensitizing of animals
with simple chemical compounds. XII. The influence of excision of
allergenic depots on onset of delayed hypersensitivity and tolerance. J.
Exp. Med. *129*, 103-121.

Magnusson, B., and Kligman, A. M. (1969). The identification of contact allergens by animal assay. The guinea pig maximization test. J. Invest. Derm. *52*, 268-276.

Magnusson, B., and Kligman, A. M. (1970). *Allergic Contact Dermatitis in the Guinea Pigs. Identification of Contact Allergens.* A. C. Thomas Publishing Co., Springfield.

Maguire, H. C. (1973). The bioassay of contact allergens in the guinea pig. J. Soc. Cosmet. Chem. *24*, 151-162.

Maibach, H., ed. (1975). *Animal Models in Dermatology. Relevance to Human Dermatopharmacology and Dermatotoxicology.* Churchill Livingstone, Edinburgh.

Malmgren, R. A., Holmes, E. C., Morton, D. L., Yee, C. L., Marrone, J., and Myers, M. W. (1969). In vitro detection of guinea pigs alloantigens by the macrophage-inhibition technique. Transplantation *8*, 485-489..

Mantoux, C. (1910). L'intradermo-réaction à la tuberculine et son interprétation clinique. Presse Med. *18*, 10-13.

Marchalonis, J. J. (1975). Lymphocyte surface immunoglobulins. Science *190*, 20-29.

Marchalonis, J. J., Bucana, C., Hoyer, L., Warr, G. W., Hanna, M. G., and Szenberg, A. (1978). Visualization of a guinea pig T lymphocyte surface component crossreactive with immunoglobulin. Science *199*, 433-435.

Markiewitz, K. H., and Dawson, C. R. (1965). On the isolation of the allergenically active components of the toxic principle of poison ivy. J. Org. Chem. *30*, 1610-1613.

Marzulli, F. N., and Maibach, H. I. (1976). Effects of vehicles and elicitation concentration in contact dermatitis testing. I. Experimental contact sensitization in humans. contact Dermatitis *2*, 325-329.

Mason, H. S., and Lada, A. (1954). Allergenic principles of poison ivy. VIII. Immunological properties of a hydrourushiol-albumin conjugate. J. Invest. Derm. *22*, 457-461.

Mason, H. S. (1955). Reactions between quinones and proteins. Nature *175*, 771-772.

Mathews, K. P., Pan, P. M., and Wells, J. H. (1972). Experience with lymphocyte transformation tests in evaluating allergy to aminosalicylic acid, isoniazid acid and streptomycin. Int. Arch. Allergy Appl. Immunol. *42*, 653-667.

Maurer, P. H., Pinchuck, P., and Gerulat, B. F. (1965). Antigenicity of polypeptides (poly alpha amino acids). XIV. Studies on immunological tolerance with structurally related synthetic polymers. Proc. Soc. Exp. Biol. Med. *118*, 1113-1118.

Maurer, T., Thomann, P., Weirich, E. G., and Hess, R. (1975). The optimization test in the guinea pig. A method for the predictive evaluation of the contact allergenicity of chemicals. Agents and Actions *5*, 174-179.

Maurer, T., Thomann, P., Weirich, E. G., and Hess, R. (1978). Predictive evaluation in animals of the contact allergenic potential of medically important substances. Part I. Comparison of different methods of inducing and measuring cutaneous sensitization. Contact Dermatitis *4*, 321-333.

Maurer, T., Thomann, P., Weirich, E. G., and Hess, R. (1979). Predictive evaluation in animals of the contact allergenic potential of medically important substances. Part II. Comparison of different methods of cutaneous sensitization with "weak" allergens. Contact Dermatitis *5*, 1-10.

Mayer, R. L. (1928). Die Uberempfindlichkeit gegen Körper von Chinonstruktur. Arch. Derm. Syph. (Berlin) *156*, 331-354.

Mayer, R. L. (1930). Untersuchugen über die durch aromatische Amine bedigten gewerblichen Erkranküngen. Arch. Gewerbepath. Gewerbehyg. *1*, 436-495.

Mayer, R. L. (1950). Compound of quinone structure as allergens and cancerogenic agents. Experientia *6*, 241-280.

McCallum, D. I. (1957). Histopathology of patch tests. Trans. St. John's Hosp. Derm. Soc. *39*, 11-19.

McCluskey, R. T., Benacerraf, B., and McCluskey, J. W. (1963). Studies on the specificity of the cellular infiltrate in delayed hypersensitivity reactions. J. Immunol. *90*, 466-477.

McDevitt, H. O., and Sela, M. (1965). Genetic control of the antibody response. I. Demonstration of determinant-specific differences in response to synthetic polypeptide antigens in two strain of inbred mice. J. Exp. Med. *122*, 517-531.

McDevitt, H. O., and Tyan, M. L. (1968). Genetic control of the antibody response in inbred mice. Transfer of response by spleen cells and linkage to the major histocompatibility (H-2) locus. J. Exp. Med. *128*, 1-11.

McFarland, W., and Heilman, D. H. (1966). Comparison of lymphocyte transformation and intradermal reactions to tuberculins. Am. Rev. Respirat. Diseases *93*, 742-748.

McFarlin, D. E., and Balfour, B. (1973). Contact sensitivity in the pig. Immunology *25*, 995-1009.

Medawar, P. B. (1965). Transplantation of tissues and organs: Introduction. Brit. Med. Bull. *21*, 97-99.

Melnick, H. D. (1971). Inhibition of macrophage migration and the mediation of cellular immunity: A review. Ann. Allergy *29*, 195-208.

Meltzer, L., and Baer, R. L. (1949). Sensitization to monoglycerol para-aminobenzoate. J. Invest. Derm. *12*, 31-39.

Miller, J. F. A. P., and Mitchell, G. F. (1968). Cell to cell interaction in the immune response. I. Hemolysin-forming cells in neonatally thymectomized mice reconstituted with thymus or thoracic duct lymphoctyes. J. Exp. Med. *128*, 801-820.

Miller, J. F. A. P., and Mitchell, G. F. (1969). Thymus and antigen-reactive cells. Transplant. Rev. *1*, 3-42.

Miller, J. F. A. P. (1971). Interaction between thymus-dependent (T) cells and bone marrow-derived (B) cells in antibody responses, in *Cell Interactions and Receptor Antibodies. Proceedings of the Third Siarid Juselius Symposium.* Mäkelä, O., Cross, A. and Kosunen, T. U., eds. Academic Press, London, pp. 293-309.

Miller, J. F. A. P., Basten, A., Sprent, J., and Cheers, C. (1971). Interaction between lymphocytes in immune responses. Cell. Immunol. *2*, 469-495.

Mills, J. A. (1966). The immunologic significance of antigen-induced lymphocyte transformation in vitro. J. Immunol. *97*, 239-247.

Milner, J. E. (1970). In vitro lymphocyte responses in contact hypersensitivity. J. Invest. Derm. *55*, 34-38.

Milner, J. E. (1971). In vitro lymphocyte responses in contact hypersensitivity. II. J. Invest. Derm. *56*, 349-352.

Milner, J. E. (1972). In vitro lymphocyte responses in contact hypersensitivity. III. J. Invest. Derm. *58*, 388-391.

Milner, J. E. (1974). In vitro lymphocyte responses in contact hypersensitivity. IV. J. Invest. Derm. *62*, 591-594.

Minamikawa, T., Jyasankar, N. P., Bohm, B. A., Taylor, I. E. P., and Towers, G. H. N. (1970). An inducible hydrolase from *Aspergillus niger,* acting on carbon-carbon bonds, for phlorrhizin and other C-alkylated phenols. Biochem. J. *116*, 889-897.

Mirza, M., Perera, M. G., and Bernstein, I. L. (1974). Leukocyte migration inhibition in nickel dermatitis. Fed. Proc. *33*, 728.

Mitchell, G. F., and Miller, J. F. A. P. (1968). Cell to cell interaction in the immune response. II. The source of hemolysin-forming cells in irradiated mice given bone marrow and thymus or thoracic duct lymphocytes. J. Exp. Med. *128*, 821-837.

Mitchell, G. F., Mishell, R. I., and Herzenberg, L. A. (1971). Studies on the influence of T cells in antibody production. Prog. Immunol. *1*, 323-335.

Mitchell, J. C. (1965). Allergy to lichens: Allergic contact dermatitis from usnic acid produced by lichenized fungi. Arch. Derm. *92*, 142-145.

Mitchell, J. C. (1966). Stereoisomeric specificity of usnic acid in delayed hypersensitivity. J. Invest. Derm. *47*, 167-168.

Mitchell, J. C., and Shibata, S. (1969). Immunologic activity of some substance derived from lichenized fungi. J. Invest. Derm. *52*, 517-520.

Mitchell, J. C., Fritig, B., Singh, B., and Towers, G. H. N. (1970). Allergic contact dermatitis from *Frullania* and *Compositae*. J. Invest. Derm. *54*, 233-239.

Mitchell, J. C., Geissman, T. A., Dupuis, G., and Towers, G. H. N. (1971). Allergic contact dermatitis causes by *Artemisia* and *Chrysanthemum* species. The role of sesquiterpene lactones. J. Invest. Derm. *56*, 98-101.

Mitchell, J. C., and Dupuis, G. (1971). Allergic contact dermatitis from sesquiterpenoids of the Compositae family of plants. Brit. J. Derm. *84*, 139-150.

Mitchell, J. C., Dupuis, G., and Geissman, T. A. (1972). Allergic contact dermatitis from sesquiterpenoids of plants. Additional allergic sesquiterpene lactones and immunological specificity of Compositae, liverwort and lichens. Brit. J. Derm. *87*, 235-240.

Mitchell, J. C. (1975). The angry back syndrome: Eczema creates eczema. Contact Dermatitis *1*, 193-194.

Mitchell, J. C. (1977). Multiple concomitant positive patch test reactions. Contact Dermatitis *3*, 315-320.

Mitchison, N. A., Rajewsky, K., and Taylor, R. B. (1970). Cooperation of antigenic determinants and of cells in the induction of antibody, in *Developmental Aspects of Antibody Formation and Structure*. Sterzl, J. and Riha, I., eds. Academic Press, New York, pp. 457-573.

Mitchison, N. A. (1971a). Carrier effect in the secondary response to hapten-proteins conjugates. I. Measurement of the effect with transferred cells and objections to the local environment hypothesis. Eur. J. Immunol. *1*, 10-17.

Mitchison, N. A. (1971b). Carrier effect in the secondary response to hapten-protein conjugates. II. Cellular cooperation. Eur. J. Immunol. *1*, 18-24.

Möller, E., Sjöberg, O., and Mäkelä, O. (1971). Immunological unresponsiveness against the (4-hydroxy-3,5-dinitrophenyl) acetyl (NNP) hapten in different lymphoid cell populations. Eur. J. Immunol. *1*, 218-220.

Möller, E., and Mäkelä, O. (1972). Antigen binding cells in immune and - tolerant mice, in *Cell Interactions, Third Lepetit Colloquium*. Silvestri, L. G., ed. North-Holland Publishing Co., Amsterdam, pp. 214-228.

Moorhead, J. W., Walters, C. S., and Claman, H. N. (1973). Immunologic reactions to haptens on autologous carriers. I. Participation of both thymus-derived and bone marrow-derived cells in the secondary in vitro response. J. Exp. Med. *137*, 411-423.

Morris, G. E. (1960). Dermatoses from phenyl-mercuric salts. Arch. Environm. Health *1*, 53-55.

Mozes, E. (1974). Cellular and molecular analysis of genetic control of the immune response in mice, in *Progress in Immunology. II.* Volume 2, Brent, L., and Holborow, J., eds. North-Holland Publishing Co. Amsterdam, pp. 191-201.

Najarian, J. S., and Feldman, J. D. (1961). Passive transfer of tuberculin sensitivity by tritiated thymidine-labelled lymphoid cells. J. Exp. Med. *114,* 779-789.

Nakagawa, S., and Tanioku, K. (1972). The induction of delayed sensitivity to 2,4-dinitrophenyl conjugates in guinea pigs sensitized with DNCB. Dermatologica *144,* 19-26.

Nathan, D. F., Karnovsky, M. L., and David, J. R. (1971). Alterations of macrophage functions by mediators from lymphocytes. J. Exp. Med. *133,* 1356-1376.

Nauciel, C., and Raynaud, M. (1971). Delayed hypersensitivity to azobenzenearsonate-*N*-acetyl-L-tyrosine. In vivo and in vitro study. Eur. J. Immunol. *1,* 257-262.

Nauciel, C. (1972). Delayed hypersensitivity to azobenzenearsonate amino acids conjugates. In vitro study of the specificity of the immune response by ^{3}H-thymidine incorporation into lymph node cells. Cell. Immunol. *5,* 587-592.

Neumann, N. P., Moore, S., and Stein, W. H. (1962). Modification of the methionine residues in ribonuclease. Biochemistry *1,* 68-75.

Nishioka, K., Aoki, T., Nishioka, K., and Tashiro, M. (1971). Studies on carrier substances of DNCB contact allergy. Dermatologica *142,* 232-240.

Nitti, F., Bovet, D., and de Pierre, F. (1937). Les phénomènes allergiques provoqués par certaines amines aromatiques. Rev. Immunol. (Paris) *3,* 376-386.

Nobréus, N., Magnusson, B., Leander, L., and Attström, R., (1974). Induction of dinitrochlorobenzene contact sensitivity in dogs. Transfer of sensitivity by thoracic duct lymphocytes and suppression of sensitivity by antithymocyte serum. Monogr. Allergy, *8,* 100-109.

Nordqvist, B., and Rorsman, H. (1967). Leukocytic migration in vitro as an indicator of allergy in eczematous contact dermatitis. Trans. Annual. Rep. St John's Hosp. Derm. Soc. *53,* 154-159.

Nossal, G. J. V., Cunningham, A., Mitchell, G. F., and Miller, J. F. A. P. (1968). Cell to cell interaction in the immune response. III. Chromosomal marker analysis of single antibody-forming cells in reconstituted, irradiated or thymectomized mice. J. Exp. Med. *128,* 839-853.

Nossal, G. J. V., and Pike, B. L. (1973). Studies on the differentiation of B lymphocytes in the mouse. Immunology *25,* 33-45.

Novogrodsky, A., and Katchalsky, E. (1971). Induction of lymphocyte transformation by periodate. FEBS Letters *12,* 297-300.

Novogrodsky, A., and Katchalski, E. (1973). Induction of lymphocyte transformation by sequential treatment with neuraminidase and galactose oxidase. Proc. Natl. Acad. Sci. U.S. *70*, 1824-1827.

Nowell, P. C. (1960). Phytohemagglutinin: An initiator of mitosis in cultures of normal human leukocytes. Cancer Res. *20*, 462-466.

Ohno, M., and Witkop, B. (1970). Cyclization of tryptophan and tryptamine derivatives to 2,3-dihydropyrrolo [2,3-*b*] indoles. J. Am. Chem. Soc. *92*, 343-348.

Ong, E. B., Shaw, E., and Schoellmann, G. (1965). The identification of the histidine residue at the active center of chymotrypsin. J. Biol. Chem. *240*, 694-698.

Oppenheim, J. J. (1968). Relationship of in vitro lymphocytes transformation to delayed hypersensitivity in guinea pigs and man. Fed. Proc. *27*, 21-28.

Oppenheim, J. J., Leventhal, B. G., and Hersh, E. M. (1968). The transformation of column-purified lymphocytes with non-specific and specific antigenic stimuli. J. Immunol. *101*, 262-270.

Ovary, Z., and Benacerraf, B. (1963). Immunological specificity of the secondary response with dinitrophenylated proteins. Proc. Soc. Exp. Biol. Med. *114*, 72-76.

Paraskevas, F., Lee, S. T., Orr, K. B., and Israels, L. G. (1972). A receptor for Fc on mouse B-lymphocytes. J. Immunol. *108*, 1319-1327.

Parker, D., Aoki, T., and Turk, J. L. (1970). Studies on the ability of the soluble proteins from skin, painted in vivo with DNFB, to cause contact sensitivity in the guinea pig. Int. Arch. Allergy Appl. Immunol. *37*, 440-448.

Parker, D., and Turk, J. L. (1970). Studies on the ability of the sub-cellular fractions of epidermis, painted in vivo with DNFB, to cause contact sensitization in the guinea pig. Int. Arch. Allergy Appl. Immunol. *37*, 440-448.

Parker, D., and Turk, J. L., ed. (1974). Contact hypersensitivity in experimental animals, in *Monographs in Allergy,* Volume 8. S. Karger, Basel.

Paul, W. E., Katz, D. H., Goidl, E. A., and Benacerraf, B. (1970). Carrier function in anti-hapten immune responses. II. Specific properties of carrier cells capable of enhancing anti-hapten antibody responses. J. Exp. Med. *132*, 283-299.

Paul, W. E. (1973). Antigen recognition and cell-receptor sites, in *Defence and Recognition,* MTP International Review of Science, Biochemistry Series One, Volume 10. Porter, R. R., ed. Butterworths, London, pp. 329-359.

Pauling, L. (1960). *The Nature of the Chemical Bond,* Third Edition. Cornell University Press, New York.

Pearmain, G., Lycette, R. R., and Fitzgerald, P. H. (1963). Tuberculin-induced mitosis in peripheral blood leukocytes. Lancet *i*, 637-638.

Perey, D. Y. E., Cooper, M. D., and Good, R. A. (1968). Lymphoepithelial tissues of the intestine and differentiation of antibody production. Science *161*, 265-266.

Perey, D. Y. E., Dupuy, J. M., and Good, R. A. (1970). Effector mechanisms of skin homograft rejection in agammaglobulinemic chickens. Transplantation *9*, 8-17.

Peterson, R. D. A., Cooper, M. D., and Good, R. A. (1965). The pathogenesis of immunologic deficiency diseases. Am. J. Med. *38*, 579-604.

Pierce, C. W., Kapp, J. A., Wood, D. D., and Benacerraf, B. (1974). Immune response in vitro. X. Functions of macrophages. J. Immunol. *112*, 1181-1189.

Pirilä, V. (1954). On the role of chrome and other trace elements in cement eczema. Acta dermato-venereol. *34*, 136-143.

Pleau, J. M., Dardenne, M., Blouquit, Y., and Bach, J. F. (1977). Structural study of circulating thymic factor: A peptide isolated from pig serum. II. Amino acid sequence. J. Biol. Chem. *252*, 8045-8047.

Polak, L., and Frey, J. R. (1973). Studies on contact hypersensitivity to chromium in the guinea pig. Inhibition of the migration of macrophages by chromium salts. Int. Arch. Allergy Appl. Immunol. *44*, 51-61.

Polak, L., Polak-Wyss, A., and Frey, J. R. (1974). Development of contact sensitivity to DNFB in guinea pigs genetically differing in their response to DNP-skin protein conjugates. Int. Arch. Allergy Appl. Immunol. *46*, 417-426.

Polak, L. (1977). Immunological aspects of contact sensitivity, in *Advances in Modern Toxicology*, Volume 4. Marzulli, F. N., and Maibach, M. I., eds. Hemisphere Publishing Corp., Washington, pp. 225-288.

Polak, L. (1980). Immunological aspects of contact sensitivity. An experimental study, in *Monographs in Allergy*, Volume 15. S. Karger AG, Basel, pp. 1-170.

Raff, M. C. (1969). Theta isoantigen as a marker of thymus derived lymphocytes in mice. Nature *224*, 378-379.

Raff, M. C. (1970a). Role of thymus-derived lymphocytes in the secondary humoral immune response in mice. Nature *226*, 1257-1258.

Raff, M. C. (1970b). Two distinct populations of peripheral lymphocytes in mice distinguishable by immunofluorescence. Immunology *19*, 637-650.

Raff, M. C., and Wortis, H. H. (1970). Thymus dependence of theta-bearing cells in the peripheral lymphoid tissues of mice. Immunology *18*, 931-942.

Raff, M. C. (1973). T and B lymphocytes and immune responses. Nature *242*, 19-23.

Rathburn, W. E., and Hildemann, W. H. (1970). Genetic control of the antibody response to simple haptens in congenic strains of mice. J. Immunol. *105*, 98-107.

Reeve, W., and Sadle, A. (1950). The reaction of propylene oxide with methanol. J. Am. Chem. Soc. *72*, 1251-1254.

Remold, H. G., Katz, A. B., Haber, E., and David, J. R. (1970). Studies on migration inhibitory factor (MIF). Recovery of MIF activity after purification by gel filtration and disc electrophoresis. Cell. Immunol. *1*, 133-145.

Richardson, W. P., and Paterson, P. Y. (1973). On the transfer of DNP-BSA hypersensitivity in guinea pigs by means of irradiated donor plasma. Evidence that the cutaneous reactivity is hapten-specific and mediated via DNP-antibody. J. Immunol. *110*, 905-910.

Ritz, H. L., Connor, D. S., and Sauter, E. D. (1975). Contact sensitization of guinea-pigs with unsaturated and halogenated sultones. Contact Dermatitis *1*, 349-358.

Rocklin, R. E., Reardon, G., Sheffer, A., Churchill, W. H., and David, J. R. (1970). Dissociation between two in vitro correlates of delayed hypersensitivity: Absence of migration inhibitory factor (MIF) in the presence of antigen-induced incorporation of ^{3}H-thymidine, in *Proceedings of the Fifth Leukocyte Culture Conference*. Harris, J. E., ed. Academic Press, New York, pp. 639-645.

Rocklin, R. E. (1973). Production of migration inhibitory factor by non-dividing lymphocytes. J. Immunol. *110*, 674-678.

Rodriguez, E., Towers, G. H. N., and Mitchell, J. C. (1976). Biological activities of sesquiterpene lactones. Phytochemistry *15*, 1573-1580.

Roed-Petersen, J., and Hjorth, N. (1976). Contact dermatitis from antioxidants. Hidden sensitizers in topical medication and foods. Brit. J. Derm. *94*, 233-241.

Roitt, I. M., Greaves, M. F., Torrigiani, G., Brostoff, J., and Playfair, J. H. L. (1969). The cellular basis of immunological responses. Lancet *11*, 367-371.

Rosenstreich, D. L., Blake, A. S., and Rosenthal, A. S. (1971). The peritoneal exudate lymphocyte. I. Difference in antigen responsiveness between peritoneal exudate and lymph node lymphocytes from immunized guinea pigs. J. Exp. Med. *134*, 1170-1187.

Rosenstreich, D. L., and Rosenthal, A. S. (1974). Peritoneal exudate lymphocyte. III. Dissociation of antigen-reactive lymphocytes from antigen-binding cells in a T lymphocyte enriched population in the guinea pig. J. Immunol. *112*, 1085-1093.

Rostenberg, A., and Haeberlin, J. B. (1950). Studies in eczematous sensitization. III. The development in species other than man or the guinea pig. J. Invest. Derm. *15*, 233-247.

Rubin, B., Schirrmacher, V., and Wigzell, H. (1973). The immune response against hapten autologous protein conjugates in the mouse. II. Carrier specificity in the secondary anti-hapten response and evidence of the existence of specific helper cells. Scand. J. Immunol. *2*, 189-197.

Rüde, E., and Günther, E. (1974). Genetic control of the immune response to synthetic polypeptide in rats and mice, in *Progress in Immunology. II. Biologic Aspects,* Volume 2. Brent, L., and Hoborow, J., eds. North-Holland Publishing Co., Amsterdam, pp. 223-233.

Saentz, A. (1938). Caractères de l'allergie et de l'immunité conférées en cobaye par l'inoculation de bacilles morts enrobés dans l'huile de vaseline. Ann. Institut Pasteur *60*, 58-94.

Salinas, M., and Subiza, E. (1956). Nuevas aportes en el canocimiento de las dermatitis por el cemento. Importancia des los iones metalicos cromo, niquel y cobalto como factores especificos sensibilizantes. Med. Segur. Trab. *4*, 13-23.

Salvin, S. B., and Smith, R. F. (1961). The specificity of allergic reactions, III. Contact hypersensitivity. J. Exp. Med. *114*, 185-194.

Sarkany, I., and Caron, G. A. (1966). Onset of antigen-induced lymphocyte transformation following smallpox vaccination. Brit. J. Derm. *78*, 352-354.

Schechter, I. (1968). Antigenic competition between polypeptidyl determinants in normal and tolerant rabbits. J. Exp. Med. *127*, 237-250.

Schlesinger, M., and Yron, I. (1969). Antigenic changes in lymph node cells after administration of antiserum to thymus cells. Science *164*, 1412-1413.

Schlesinger, M. (1970). Anti-theta antibodies for detecting thymus-dependent lymphocytes in the immune response of mice to SRBC. Nature *226*, 1254-1256.

Schlesinger, D. H., Goldstein, G., and Niall, H. D. (1975). The complete amino acid sequence of ubiquitin, an adenylate cyclase stimulating polypeptide probably universal in living cells. Biochemistry *12*, 2214-2218.

Schlesinger, D. H., and Goldstein, G. (1975). The amino acid sequence of thymopoietin. II. Cell *5*, 361-365.

Schlewer, G., Stampf, J. L., and Benezra, C. (1978). Synthesis of and allergic contact dermatitis to bicyclo-[2,2,1]-1-heptyl-α-methylene-γ-butyrolactones derived from norbornene and camphene. Can. J. Biochem. *56*, 153-157.

Schlewer, G., Stampf, J. L., and Benezra, C. (1980a). Synthesis of α-methyl-α-butyrolactones: Structure-activity relationships and study of their allergenic power. J. Med. Chem. *23*, 1031-1038.

Schlewer, G., Benezra, C., Beck, G., and Beck, J. P. (1980b). The cytotoxic properties of α-mono-β,α and α,α-disubstituted α-methylene-γ-butyrolactones. Toxicol. Eur. Res. *II*, 223-226.

Schlossman, S. F., Yaron, A., Ben-Efraim, S., and Sober, H. A. (1965). Immunogenicity of a series of α,N-DNP-lysines. Biochemistry *4*, 1638-1645.

Schlossman, S. F., Ben-Efraim, S., Yaron, A., and Sober, H. A. (1966). Immunochemical studies on the antigenic determinants required to elicit delayed and immediate hypersensitivity reactions. J. Exp. Med. *123*, 1083-1085.

Schlossman, S. F., and Levine, H. (1967). Immunochemical studies on delayed and Arthus-type hypersensitivity reactions. I. The relationship between antigenic determinant size and antibody combining site size. J. Immunol. *98*, 211-219.

Schlossman, S. F., and Yaron, A. (1970). Immunochemical studies on the specificity of cellular and antibody-mediated immune reactions. Ann. N.Y. Acad. Sci. *169*, 108-115.

Schoellmann, G., and Shaw, E. (1963). Direct evidence for the presence of histidine in the active center of chymotrypsin. Biochemistry *2*, 252-255.

Schulz, K. H. (1960). Gruppenallergie gegenüber Thioglykolsaürederivaten. Arch. Klin. Exp. Derm. *211*, 253-260.

Schwartz, L., Tulipan, L., and Peck, S. M. (1948). *Occupational Diseases of the Skin.* Lea and Febiger, Philadelphia.

Schwarzschild, L. (1928). Sensibilisierung aus der Orthoformreihe. Arch. Derm. Syph. (Berlin) *156*, 432-445.

Sefik, S. A., Williams, E. B., Nitecki, E. E., and Goodman, J. W. (1972). Antigen recognition and the immune response. Humoral and cellular immune responses to small mono- and bifunctional antigen molecules. J. Exp. Med. *135*, 1228-1246.

Seidmann, M. (1946). Dermatitis among workers employed in the citrus by-product industry. Harefuah *2*, 39-49.

Sela, M., and Arnon, R. (1960). Studies on the chemical basis of the antigenicity of proteins. Biochem. J. *75*, 91-102.

Sela, M. (1966). Immunological studies with synthetic polypeptides. Adv. Immunol. *5*, 29-129.

Sell, S., and Gell, P. G. H. (1965). Studies on rabbit lymphocytes in vitro. I. Stimulation of blast transformation with an antiallotype serum. J. Exp. Med. *122*, 423-440.

Sharon, N., and Lis, H. (1972). Lectins: Cell agglutinating and sugar-specific proteins. Science *177*, 949-959.

Shaw, E., Mares-Guia, M., and Cohen, W. (1965). Evidence for an active-center histidine in trypsin through use of a specific reagent. 1-Chloro-3-tosylamino-7-amino-2-heptatone, the chloromethylketone derived from N,α-tosyl-L-lysine. Biochemistry *4*, 2219-2224.

Shevach, E. M., Jaffe, E. S., and Green, I. (1973). Receptor for complement and immunoglobulin on human and animal lymphoid cells. Transplant. Rev. *16*, 3-28.

Shigeno, N., Arpels, C., Hammerling, U., Boyse, E. A., and Old, L. J. (1968). Preparation of lymphocyte-specific antibody from antilymphocyte serum. Lancet *ii*, 320-323.

Shortman, K., Diener, E., Russell, P., and Armstrong, W. D. (1970). The role of nonlymphoid accessory cells in the immune response to different antigens. J. Exp. Med. *131*, 461-482.

Shortman, K., and Palmer, J. (1971). The requirement for macrophages in the immune response in vitro. Cell. Immunol. *2*, 399-410.

Shmunes, E., Katz, S. A., and Samitz, M. H. (1973). Chromium-amino acid conjugates as elicitors in chromium sensitized guinea pigs. J. Invest. Derm. *60*, 193-196.

Sidi, E., Hindky, J., and Hindky, M. (1964). Le rôle de la constitution chimique dans les allergies de contact. Rev. franc. Allergie *4*, 1-19.

Silberberg, I. (1971). Ultrastructural studies of Langerhans cells in contact sensitive and primary irritant reactions to mercuric chloride. Clin. Research *19*, 715.

Silberberg, I., Baer, R. L., and Rosenthal, S. A. (1974a). Circulating Langerhans cells in a dermal vessel. Acta Dermato-Venereol. *54*, 81-86.

Silberberg, I., Baer, R. L., and Rosenthal, S. A. (1974b). The role of Langerhans cells in contact allergy. I. An ultrastructural study in actively induced contact dermatitis in guinea pigs. Acta Dermato-Venereol. *54*, 321-331.

Silberberg, I., Baer, R. L., Rosenthal, S. A., Thorbecke, G. J., and Berezowsky, V. (1975). Dermal and intravascular Langerhans cells at sites of passively induced allergic contact sensitivity. Immunology *18*, 435-453.

Silberberg, I., Baer, R. L., and Rosenthal, S. A. (1976). The role of Langerhans cells in allergic contact hypersensitivity. A review of finding in man and guinea pigs. J. Invest. Derm. *66*, 210-217.

Silverstein, A. M., and Gell, P. G. H. (1962). Delayed hypersensitivity to hapten-protein conjugates. II. Anti hapten specificity and the heterogeneity of the delayed response. J. Exp. Med. *115*, 1053-1064.

Snell, G. D., Cherry, M., McKenzie, I. F. C., and Bailey, D. W. (1973). Ly-4, a new locus determining a lymphocyte cell-surface alloantigen in mice. Proc. Natl. Acad. Sci. U.S. *70,* 1108-1111.

Sprent, J., and Miller, J. F. A. P. (1972a). Interaction of thymus lymphocytes with histoincompatible cells. I. Quantitation of the proliferative response of thymus cells. Cell. Immunol. *3,* 361-384.

Sprent, J., and Miller, J. F. A. P. (1972b). Interaction of thymus lymphocytes with histocompatible cells. III. Immunological characteristics of recirculating lymphocytes derived from activated thymus cells. Cell. Immunol. *3,* 213-230.

Stampf, J. L., Schlewer, G., Ducombs, G., Foussereau, J., and Benezra, C. (1978). Allergic contact dermatitis due to sesquiterpene lactones. A comparative study of human and animal sensitivity to α-methylene-γ-butyrolactone and derivatives. Brit. J. Derm. *99,* 163-169.

Storck, H., and Schwarz, M. (1960). Observations on allergenicity of simple inorganic compounds. Acta allergologica. Suppl. VII. 232-239.

Storck, H. (1962). Das experimentelle Ekzem, in *Handbuch der Haut und Geschlechtskrankheiten.* Jadassohn, J., ed. Erganzungswerk II/I. Springer-Verlag, Berlin, pp. 113-211.

St-Rose, J. E. M., and Cinader, B. (1967). The effect of tolerance on the specificity of the antibody response and on immunogenicity. Antibody response to conformationally and chemically altered antigens. J. Exp. Med. *125,* 1031-1055.

Strauss, H. W. (1937). Studies in experimental hypersensitiveness in the rhesus monkey. I. Active sensitization with poison ivy. J. Immunol. *32,* 241-249.

Subba Rao, P. V., Mangala, A., Towers, G. H. N., and Rodriguez, E. (1978). Immunological activity of parthenin and its diastereoisomer in persons sensitized by *Parthenium hysterophobus L.* Contact Dermatitis *4,* 199-203.

Sulzberger, M. B., and Baer, R. L. (1938). Sensitization to simple chemicals. III. Relationship between chemical structure and properties, and sensitizing capacities in the production of eczematous sensitivity in man. J. Invest. Derm. *1,* 45-48.

Symes, W. F., and Dawson, C. R. (1954). Poison ivy urushiol. J. Am. Chem. Soc. *76,* 2959-2963.

Tanford, C. (1973). *The Hydrophobic Effect.* Wiley-Interscience Publication, New York.

Taugner, M., and Schültz, R. (1966). Beitrage zur Quecksilber-Allergie. Dermatologica *133,* 245-261.

Taylor, R. B. (1969). Cellular cooperation in the antibody response of mice to two serum albumins: Specific function of thymus cells. Transplant. Rev. *1,* 114-149.

Thulin, H., and Zacharinae, H. (1972). The leukocyte migration test in chromium hypersensitivity. J. Invest. Derm. *58*, 55-58.

Trainin, N., Small, M., Zipori, D., Umiel, T., Kook, A. I., and Rotter, U. (1975a). Characteristics of THF, a thymic hormone, in *Biological Activity of Thymic Hormones*. Van Bekhum, D. W., and Kruisbeek, A. M., eds. Kooyker Scientific Publications, Rotterdam, pp. 117-144.

Trainin, N., Kook, A. I., Umiel, T., and Albala, M. (1975b). The nature and mechanism of stimulation of immune responsiveness by thymus extract. Ann. N.Y. Acad. Sci. *249,* 349-361.

Turk, J. L. (1962). The passive transfer of delayed hypersensitivity in guinea pigs by the transfusion of isotopically labelled lymphoid cells. Immunol. *5,* 478-488.

Turk, J. L., and Oort, J. (1963). A histological study of the early stages of the development of the tuberculin reaction after passive transfer of cells labelled with ^{3}H-thymidine. Immunology *6,* 140-147.

Turk, J. L., and Stone, S. M. (1963). Implications of the cellular changes in lymph nodes during the development and inhibition of delayed type hypersensitivity, in *Cell-Bound Antibodies*. Amos, B. and Koprowsky, H., eds. Wistar Institute Press, Philadelphia, pp. 51-54.

Turk, J. L., Rudner, E. J., and Heather, C. J. (1966). A histochemical analysis of mononuclear cell infiltrates of the skin. II. Delayed hypersensitivity in the human. Int. Arch. Allergy Appl. Immunol. *30,* 248-256.

Turk, J. L., and Oort, J. (1970). The production of sensitized cells in cell-mediated immunity, in *Handbuch der allgemeinen Pathologie,* Volume VII. Studer, A., and Cottier, H., eds. Springer-Verlag, Berlin, pp. 392-435.

Turk, J. L. (1975). Delayed hypersensitivity, in *Frontiers of Biology*, Second revised edition. Neuberger, A., and Tatum, E. L., eds. North-Holland Publishing Co., Amsterdam.

Uhr, J. W., and Phillips, J. M. (1966). In vitro sensitization of phagocytes and lymphocytes by antigen-antibody complexes. Ann. N.Y. Acad. Sci. *129,* 793-798.

Uhr, J. W., and Vitetta, E. S. (1973). Synthesis, biochemistry and dynamics of cell surface immunoglobulin on lymphocytes. Fed. Proc. *32,* 35-40.

Unanue, E. R., Engers, H. D., and Karnovsky, M. J. (1973). Antigen receptors on lymphocytes. Fed. Proc. *32,* 44-47.

Valdimarsson, H., Higgs, J. M., Wells, P. S., Yamamura, M., Hobbs, J. R., and Holt, P. J. (1973). Immune abnormalities associated with chronic mucocutaneous candidiasis. Cell. Immunol. *6,* 348-361.

Van Lier, J. E., and Smith, L. L. (1970). Autoxidation of cholesterol via hydroperoxide intermediates. J. Org. Chem. *35,* 2627-2632.

Vickers, H. R. (1941). The carrot as a cause of dermatitis. Brit. J. Derm. *53*, 52-57.

Waldron, G. W. (1934). Hypersensitivity to procaine. Proc. Mayo Clin. *9*, 254-256.

Walters, C. S., and Wigzell, H. (1970). Demonstration of heavy and light chain antigenic determinant on the cell bound receptor for antigen. Similarities between membrane attached and humoral antibodies produced by the same cell. J. Exp. Med. *132*, 1233-1249.

Ward, P. A., Remold, H. G., and David, J. R. (1970). The production by antigen-stimulated lymphocytes of a leukotactic factor distinct from migration inhibitory factor. Cell. Immunol. *1*, 162-174.

Waskman, B. H., and Arbouys, S. (1962). The use of specific "lymphocyte" anti-sera to inhibit hypersensitive reactions of the "delayed" type, in *Mechanisms of Antibody Formation.* Holub, M., and Jaroskova, L., eds. Academic Press, New York, pp. 165-178.

Watson, J., Thoman, M., Ralph, P., and Trenkner, E. (1974). The role of humoral factors in the initiation of in vitro primary immune responses. IV. Are macrophages the adherent cell type required for cell cooperation? J. Immunol. *112*, 1873-1883.

Watson, J. D. (1977). *Molecular Biology of the Gene,* Third edition. W. A. Benjamin Inc., Menlo Park, California.

Wedroff, N. S. (1927). Zur Frage der Dinitrochlorbenzoldermatosen. Arch. Derm. Syph. (Berlin) *154*, 143-153.

Wedroff, N. S. (1932). Zur frage der Sensibilisierun der Haut: Die Sensibilisierung für dinitrochlorbenzol unter Gewerbebedingungen. Arch. Gewerpathol. Gewerbyg. *3*, 509-522.

Wedroff, N. S., and Dolgoff, A. P. (1935). Uber die spezifische Sensibilistal der Haut einfachen chemischen Stoffen gegenuber. Arch. Derm. Syph. (Berlin) *171*, 647-664.

Wheland, G. W., and Pauling, L. (1935). A quantum-mechanical discussion of orientation of substituents in aromatic molecules. J. Am. Chem. Soc. *57*, 2086-2095.

White, A., and Burton, P. (1979). Isolation from human plasma of a protein fraction with thymic hormone-like activity. Ann. N.Y. Acad. Sci. *332*, 1-8.

Wieghardt, T., and Goren, H. J. (1975). The reactivity of imidazole nitrogens in histidine alkylation. Bioorganic Chem. *4*, 30-40.

Wigzell, H., and Andersson, B. (1969). Cell separation on antigen-coated columns. Elimination of high rate antibody-forming cells and immunological memory cells. J. Exp. Med. *129*, 23-36.

Wilkinson, D. S., Fregert, S., Magnusson, B., Bandmann, H.-J., Calnan, C. D., Cronin, E., Hjorth, N., Maibach, H. I., Malten, K. E., Menegghi, C. L., and Pirilä, V. (1970). Acta Dermato-Venereol. *50*, 287-292.

Williams, A. (1969). Mechanism of action and specificity or proteolytic enzymes. Quart. Rev. *23*, 1-17.

Willoughby, D. A., Boughton, B., Spector, W. G., and Schild, H. O. (1962). A vascular permeability factor extracted from normal and sensitized guinea-pig lymph node cells. Life Sciences *7*, 347-252.

Wilson, D. B., Silvers, W. K., and Nowell, P. C. (1967). Quantitative studies on the mixed lymphocyte interaction in rats. II. Relationship of the proliferative response. J. Exp. Med. *126*, 655-665.

Woodward, R. B., Cava, M. P., Ollis, W. D., Hunger, A., Daeniker, H. U., and Schenker, J. (1963). The total synthesis of strychnine. Tetrahedron *19*, 247-288.

Yaron, A., Dunham, E. K., and Schlossman, S. F. (1974). Synthesis and immunological properties of the oligolysyl-N^{ϵ}-dinitrophenyllysine and oligolysyl-alanylalanylalanyl-N^{ϵ}-dinitrophenyllysine peptide series. Biochemistry *13*, 347-354.

Yoshioka, H., Mabry, T. J., and Timmermann, B. N. (1973). *Sesquiterpene Lactones*. University of Tokyo Press, Tokyo.

Zina, B., and Bonu, G. (1965). Il ruolo dei coloranti azoici come allergeni primari da contalto. Minerva Derm. *40*, 307-315.

Zinsser, H. (1925). Bacterial allergies and tissue reactions. Proc. Soc. Exp. Biol. Med. *22*, 35-39.

Zweiman, B., and Silberberg, D. H. (1971). In vitro lymphocyte responsiveness of human subjects receiving azathioprine. Int. Arch. Allergy Appl. Immunol. *41*, 428-433.

Abbreviations

ABA	azobenzenearsonate
ACD	allergic contact dermatitis
Ar	aryl (aromatic) group
BGG	bovine gammaglobulin
BHA	butylated hydroxyanisole
BHT	butylated hydroxytoluene
CFA	complete Freund's adjuvant
DDT	1,1,1-trichloro-2,2-bis(p-chlorophenyl)ethane
DES	diethylstilbestrol
DNCB	1-chloro-2,4-dinitrobenzene
DNFB	1-fluoro-2,4-dinitrobenzene
DNP	2,4-dinitrophenyl
FD&C	Federal Food, Drug and Cosmetic Act
HSA	human serum albumin
m	meta (substitution on a benzene ring)
MIF	(macrophage) migration inhibition factor
NDGA	nordihydroguaiaretic acid
o	ortho (substitution on a benzene ring)
p	para (substitution on a benzene ring)
PPD	paraphenylenediamine
SLS	sodium laurylethersulfate
TCSA	3,3',4,5'-tetrachlorosalicylanilide
TLCK	N-tosyllysinechloromethylketone
TPCK	N-tosylphenylalaninechloromethylketone

Author Index

Numbers indicate that an author's work is referred to. Italic numbers give the page on which the complete reference is listed.